How to Survive in Anaesthesia

D1355055

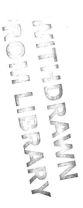

How to Survive in Anaesthesia

A guide for trainees

FOURTH EDITION

Neville Robinson

Department of Anaesthesia
Northwick Park and St Mark's Hospitals
Harrow, Middlesex
UK

George Hall

Department of Anaesthesia
St George's
University of London
London
UK

William Fawcett

Department of Anaesthesia
Royal Surrey County Hospital
Guildford, Surrey
UK

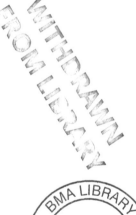

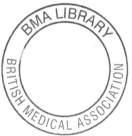

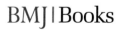

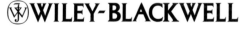

A John Wiley & Sons, Ltd., Publication

Library of Congress Cataloging-in-Publication Data

Robinson, Neville.
  How to survive in anaesthesia : a guide for trainees. – 4th ed. /
Neville Robinson, George Hall, William Fawcett.
    p. ; cm.
  Includes index.
  ISBN 978-0-470-65462-0 (pbk.)
  1. Anesthesiologists–Training of.   2. Anesthesiology–Study and teaching.   3. Anesthesia.
I. Hall, George M. (George Martin)   II. Fawcett, William, 1962-   III. Title.
  [DNLM: 1. Anesthesia–methods. WO 200]
  RD81.R655 2011
  617.9′6092–dc23   2011018481

A catalogue record for this book is available from the British Library.

This book is published in the following electronic formats: ePDF 9781119950431; Wiley Online Library 9781119950462; ePub 9781119950448

Set in 9.5/12pt Minion by Aptara Inc., New Delhi, India
Printed and bound in Malaysia by Vivar Printing Sdn Bhd

2   2013

This book is dedicated to Charlotte Fawcett

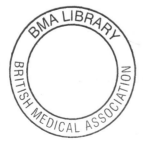

Contents

Part III: Passing the gas, 125

List of boxes

List of figures

List of tables

Preface to the fourth edition

We have updated the content for this edition and added one essential chapter. We wish to thank readers for their helpful comments, and hope that our ideal of assisting anaesthetic novices in providing safe anaesthetic skills and practice is still achieved.

William Fawcett has generously agreed to assist with authorship of the book and has provided the text with a new freshness. He has added some case studies to the clinical sections and has contributed to the content of the whole text.

Neville Robinson
George Hall
William Fawcett

Preface to the third edition

We have added two chapters in response to discussion with trainees who asked for examples of anaesthetic mishaps and help in assessing sick patients. The emphasis remains on providing an introductory text to safe clinical practice. We are grateful to our many colleagues, senior and junior, for their support and advice, particularly Neville Goodman.

Neville Robinson
George Hall

Preface to the second edition

We are grateful for the many comments received about the contents and style of the first edition. We have taken the opportunity to decrease the size of the book to make it more of a 'pocket book' and we have revised the text and added two new chapters.

Our main aim remains to provide a concise readable text that will introduce the new trainee in anaesthesia to *safe* clinical practice. In addition, the contents of the book are applicable to many clinical aspects of the primary Fellowship examination of the Royal College of Anaesthetists.

Neville Robinson
George Hall

Preface to the first edition

If you are a trained anaesthetist, you should not be reading this. If you have just started anaesthesia, congratulations on your choice; you have joined the most interesting specialty in medicine which contains some of the most intelligent, well-adjusted consultants to be found in hospitals (we can think of at least two). In your first few weeks of anaesthesia you will be given much advice, some of which may even be good, and will be influenced by the current issues affecting the specialty. It is easy to believe that audit, high dependency units, acute pain teams, *et cetera*, are areas of essential knowledge for the newcomer. They are not. They only become relevant when you are capable of conducting a safe anaesthetic. We hope that this short book will help trainees in the first year of anaesthesia by emphasising basic principles and key concepts. Full explanations have been left for 'proper' textbooks.

We thank the many trainees who over the years have kept us entertained, enthused, sometimes informed, occasionally frightened, and whose ingenuity in devising new mistakes never ceased to amaze.

Neville Robinson
George Hall

Let's start at the very beginning . . .

If you are starting as a trainee in anaesthesia with little knowledge of how operating theatres work, read this. If you understand the theatre environment, go to Chapter 1.

What you need

You will need your ID badge, two pens (one invariably runs out of ink or is borrowed), a stethoscope and a copy of this book.

Where to go

You need to find the correct changing room, male or female, and change into theatre scrubs, hat and suitable footwear. Do not leave anything valuable in your clothes; lock it away or take it with you. Do not enter the wrong changing room 'by mistake' more than once. Do not borrow theatre shoes: the pair you take will belong to one of the senior surgeons, who will make your life a misery for the next few months when (s)he finds that they are missing. Face masks are usually unnecessary except in theatres in which a prosthesis is inserted, such as orthopaedics.

You will see staff wandering round the hospital and even local shops in theatre scrubs. One author even saw a person wearing theatre scrubs in an international airport. This is inappropriate, and you should change each time you leave the operating theatres.

How to behave

You should be punctual, polite and pleasant to all theatre staff. As a new anaesthetic trainee you are at the very bottom of the theatre hierarchy.

Key people in theatres

In each operating theatre there is a scrub nurse and a runner, who is not scrubbed, who fetches instruments for the surgical team. There is usually a theatre sister in overall charge. In the UK the anaesthetist always works with a trained assistant. They may be called an operating department practitioner (ODP), operating department assistant (ODA) or anaesthetic nurse. They will have undergone at least two years of training and are often skilled in resuscitation and trauma assessment. Watch carefully how they prepare for cases and listen to any advice they may give. Very few ODPs are unhelpful to new trainees and the best are outstanding. We have learnt much from experienced ODPs and value their knowledge, commitment and friendship.

The theatre manager is an important person, so introduce yourself and try to gain their support (see *How to behave*). The theatre receptionist/secretary has to deal with the running of the theatres and is often very knowledgeable about the likes and dislikes of senior staff. Time spent in idle chat is usually time well spent.

Key people in anaesthetic departments

The most important person in the anaesthetic department is the secretary/rota organiser. You must not upset them – they can make your life miserable. Other people in the department, who think that they are important, include the College tutor, educational supervisors, module supervisors, clinical supervisors, mentors and the head of department. It is very difficult to find any consultant without a label. The longer the title, the less important the position.

You should not need to bother these people in the first few weeks. In many departments you will work with a few senior staff who will guide you gently through the basics of anaesthesia. They are chosen for their kindness, imperturbability and good humour in the presence of the chaos of your initial attempts at anaesthesia. It is their job to imprint safe anaesthetic practice into your receptive brain. You will remember them long after you have forgotten the name of the head of department.

Cleanliness and sterility

Cleanliness is important for all theatre staff. Hands must be washed, or an alcohol handrub used, before and after touching patients. This boring ritual is necessary to minimise infections acquired in theatres.

The patient's skin should be cleaned with chlorhexidine 2% in isopropyl alcohol 70% before the insertion of needles and cannulae. For central venous cannulation and neuraxial blockade the anaesthetist should adopt surgical sterility: gown, gloves, hat and mask.

Controlled drugs

The supply and use of drugs that can cause dependency or abuse, such as opioids, benzodiazepines and cocaine, is tightly controlled by law. These drugs are kept in a locked cupboard, and when they are used you must:

- sign the controlled drug register. This is countersigned by another qualified person (nurse/qualified ODP). Your signature confirms that the number of remaining ampoules is correct.
- record the amount of drug given to the patient on the anaesthetic chart.
- return unopened ampoules to the locked cupboard.
- not use the contents of an ampoule for more than one patient.
- discard any drug not used, ideally in the presence of a third party.

Although these regulations may appear onerous, they have contributed to the very low prevalence of drug dependency among anaesthetists in the UK.

Consent/WHO checklist

Anaesthesia is not overburdened with paperwork but there are two key documents that must be checked before surgery starts. The consent form, which gives details of the surgical procedure, must have been signed by the patient and witnessed by a member of the surgical team. The identity of the patient must be determined to ensure that the right patient is in the right place for the right operation.

Most hospitals have adopted the WHO Surgical Safety Checklist, which aims to prevent wrong-site surgery and decrease surgical complications. Although most of the details are surgical, the anaesthetist is asked for the ASA status of the patient (see Chapter 21) and if they have any concerns. The latter refers to medical, not personal, concerns so it is inappropriate to mention your doubts about the possible health hazards of your recent social life. All members of the theatre team are introduced by name and role, which is a rapid way of integrating new trainees.

Anaesthetic charts

The anaesthetic chart is a contemporaneous record of what happened to the patient while they were your responsibility. It is a very important document that must be completed legibly, accurately and in appropriate detail. The chart may be analysed very closely in the future by the legal profession, who will emphasise any omissions, errors and illegibility. A scruffy chart with coffee stains creates a bad impression. Anaesthetic charts vary slightly from hospital to hospital but contain the following basic information:

- patient details
- preoperative assessment
- intraoperative management
- postoperative instructions

The chart should contain enough information so that another anaesthetist could give an identical anaesthetic from the information recorded.

Enthusiasts

The senior anaesthetists who supervise your intitial training will protect you from the more eccentric members of the profession. However, you will encounter enthusiasts who believe passionately that their anaesthetic techniques are superior to those of others. Three groups are easily recognised: regional anaesthesia enthusiasts (always needing the ultrasound machine), infusion enthusiasts (the more infusion pumps the better the anaesthetic) and technology enthusiasts (always using the latest equipment with many totally unnecessary functions). They all have useful knowledge to impart but should be avoided until you can give a safe simple anaesthetic.

. . . when you read you begin with A-B-C (airway-breathing-circulation) so read on.

(with apologies to *The Sound of Music*)

Part I **Nuts and bolts**

The first section of this book deals with two fundamental aspects of anaesthetic practice: the airway and vascular access.

General anaesthesia has been summarised by the simple phrase *put up a drip, put down a tube and give plenty of oxygen.* Although many anaesthetists resent this glib description of their work, it does have the virtue of emphasising the importance of venous cannulation and control of the airway, which are essential for the safe conduct of anaesthesia. Difficulties arise in anaesthesia when one of these fundamental areas is not secure, and if both fail then disaster is close at hand.

Therefore, in the first 10 chapters we concentrate on evaluation and control of the airway, the anaesthetic machine and circuits, basic anaesthetic monitoring, vascular access, and the choice of intravenous fluids. We have not given detailed instructions on how to undertake the practical procedures.

There is no substitute for careful instruction from a senior anaesthetist as part of the anaesthetic procedure. At the start of training the application of physiology and pharmacology to anaesthesia is exciting, and knowledge of the equipment may seem mundane and even boring.

It is imperative that you have a basic understanding of the equipment you use – failure to do so will put the patient at risk.

Chapter 1 **Evaluation of the airway**

Experienced anaesthetists teach that there are three fundamental aspects to safe anaesthetic practice: the airway, the airway and the airway. Unanticipated airway problems account for about 40% of overall anaesthetic morbidity and mortality. Tracheal intubation is now undertaken less often, mainly because of the advent of supraglottic airways such as the laryngeal mask. However, tracheal intubation remains the gold standard for airway management, control and protection. It may be required during the course of an anaesthetic or for the management of an unconscious patient. Therefore, careful airway assessment must be undertaken. This is carried out logically, as summarised in Box 1.1.

Box 1.1 Assessment of the airway

- History
- Symptoms
- Examination
  - anatomy and variants
  - medical conditions
  - specific assessment
    - Mallampati scoring system
    - thyromental distance
    - sternomental distance
  - other tests

1.1 History

Any previous anaesthetic history must be obtained. Information about difficulties with tracheal intubation may be found in old anaesthetic records.

How to Survive in Anaesthesia: A Guide for Trainees, Fourth Edition.
Neville Robinson, George Hall and William Fawcett.
© 2012 John Wiley & Sons, Ltd. Published 2012 by John Wiley & Sons, Ltd.

Previous successful intubation is not an indicator of its ease. Some patients carry letters or wear MedicAlert bracelets stating their anaesthetic difficulties, while others with major problems know nothing about them. Ascertain whether the airway is potentially difficult by checking whether the patient has any of the medical and surgical conditions listed in Box 1.2.

Box 1.2 Medical features of difficult airway intubation

- Congenital: rare
- Acquired
    - traumatic: fractures of mandible and cervical spine
    - infection: epiglottitis, dental or facial abscess
    - endocrine: thyroid enlargement, acromegaly, obesity
    - neoplasia: tongue, neck, mouth, radiotherapy
    - inflammatory: ankylosing spondylitis, rheumatoid arthritis
    - pregnancy

1.2 Symptoms

Upper airway obstruction may be found in patients with stridor, dysphagia and hoarseness.

1.3 Examination and clinical tests

Normal anatomy and its variants

Some patients appear anatomically normal and yet are difficult, or impossible, to intubate. These patients cause anaesthetists unexpected problems. We have had the occasional experience of casually starting an apparently normal laryngoscopy, only to have the sinking feeling associated with complete failure to see the larynx. It is much better to anticipate a difficulty than encounter one unexpectedly. Some anatomical factors that make airway control and intubation difficult are listed in Box 1.3.

Box 1.3 Anatomical features of difficult airway control and intubation

- Short immobile neck
- Full set of teeth, buck teeth
- High arch palate
- Poor mouth opening – less than three fingers gap between upper and lower teeth

---

- Receding mandible (may be hidden by a beard)
- Inability to sublux the jaw (forward protrusion of the lower incisors beyond the upper incisors)

Specific assessment

Several clinical tests to assess the airway are in common use. None is reliable in predicting a difficult airway or intubation, and all should be used in combination as this provides a better overall assessment of the airway.

Modified Mallampati scoring system

This predicts about 50% of difficult intubations. The test can be performed with the patient in the upright or supine position. It is based upon the visibility of the pharyngeal structures with the mouth open as wide as possible (Figure 1.1). Patients are classified as follows:

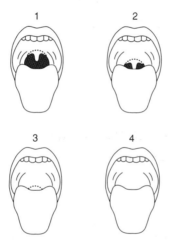

Figure 1.1 Structures seen on opening of mouth for Mallampati grades 1–4.

- Grade 1: faucial pillars, soft palate and uvula visible
- Grade 2: faucial pillars, soft palate visible, but uvula masked by the base of the tongue
- Grade 3: soft palate only visible
- Grade 4: soft palate not visible

Patients in grades 3 and 4 are considered difficult to intubate, and those in grades 1 and 2 are considered feasible intubations. It is important to realise that this system is *not* infallible, and patients in grade 2 sometimes cannot be intubated.

Head and neck movement
Flexion and extension are greater than 90° in normal people.

Jaw movement and mandible
Check that the patient's mouth opens normally. It should have an interincisor gap of greater than 5 cm (about three finger breadths). Check that the patient does not have buck teeth or a receding mandible. Ideally, the lower incisors should be able to be protruded beyond the upper incisors. If these simple tests cannot be performed the airway may be difficult to manage.

Thyromental distance
The thyromental distance (Patil test) is the distance from the thyroid cartilage to the mental prominence when the neck is extended fully (Figure 1.2). In the absence of other anatomical factors, if the distance is more than 6.5 cm, problems should not occur with intubation. A distance of less than 6 cm suggests laryngoscopy will be impossible, and for distances of 6–6.5 cm laryngoscopy is considered difficult, but possible. This measurement may predict up to 75% of difficult intubations.

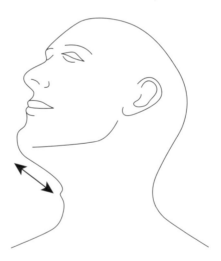

Figure 1.2 Line shows the thyromental distance from the thyroid cartilage to the tip of the chin.

Sternomental distance
This test is claimed to predict up to 90% of difficult intubations. The distance from the upper border of the manubrium sterni to the tip of the chin, with

the mouth closed and the head fully extended, is measured. A distance of less than 12.5 cm indicates a difficult intubation.

1.4 Other tests

Indirect laryngoscopy and various x-ray procedures are occasionally used. Using x-rays, the effective mandibular length is compared with the posterior depth of the mandible; a ratio of more than 3.6 may be associated with a difficult intubation. A decreased distance between the occiput and the spinous process of C1 is also reported as associated with difficulties with laryngoscopy. We have found these tests to be of limited value.

1.5 Conclusion

The airway must be assessed before any anaesthetic procedure is embarked upon. Airway control and tracheal intubation is occasionally difficult, or even impossible, in anatomically normal people. An assessment from the patient's history, symptoms and medical conditions, combined with careful clinical examination, will help avoid most, but not all, unexpectedly difficult intubations.

Chapter 2 **Control of the airway**

The novice anaesthetist must learn rapidly the skills of airway control.

2.1 Position

The patient must be correctly positioned. This is achieved by elevating the head by about the height of a pillow to flex the neck. The head is extended on the cervical spine and the mandible lifted forward to stop obstruction from the tongue and other pharyngeal structures that lose their tone under anaesthesia. This position is commonly referred to as 'sniffing the early morning air' – a practice not to be recommended in a modern urban environment.

2.2 Methods

Four methods of airway control are used to ensure unobstructed gaseous exchange (Box 2.1).

Box 2.1 Methods of airway control

- Face mask and Guedel airway
- Laryngeal mask
- Tracheal tube
- Tracheostomy

Face mask

The mask is designed to fit snugly over the patient's nose and mouth. However, gas often leaks round the side of the mask in edentulous patients. Clear masks

How to Survive in Anaesthesia: A Guide for Trainees, Fourth Edition.
Neville Robinson, George Hall and William Fawcett.
© 2012 John Wiley & Sons, Ltd. Published 2012 by John Wiley & Sons, Ltd.

allow you to see the airway and any secretions or vomit. Newer masks have inflatable rims that allow air to be added or removed from the mask to improve the tightness of the seal. An obstructed airway may be relieved by the insertion of an oropharyngeal airway (Guedel airway) or by a nasopharyngeal airway. Guedel airways are sized from 0 to 4, with a size 3 used for adult females and 4 for adult males. Nasopharyngeal airways, unless they are inserted very gently, can cause haemorrhage, which may further threaten the airway.

Laryngeal mask

This was developed from the concept that the anaesthetic face mask could, instead of being applied to the face, be altered and positioned over the laryngeal opening (Figure 2.1). It is inserted using a blind technique and provides a patent airway for spontaneous breathing. It is used increasingly for ventilation and management of difficult intubation.

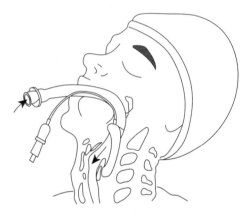

Figure 2.1 Laryngeal mask correctly positioned before inflation, with the tip of the mask in the base of the hypopharynx.

The original design of laryngeal mask was re-usable after autoclaving. There are now many disposable options available but these are often more difficult to insert. Most laryngeal mask airways require the addition of 20–30 ml of air to expand the cuff, and this provides a snug fit of the mask in the oropharynx. Some supraglottic airways come with a preformed cuff that does not require inflation. Flexible or non-kinking versions are also used. An oesophageal port is available on some tubes; this is designed to allow vomit to pass directly out of the tube, which in theory minimises tracheal contamination from the vomit. The experienced anaesthetist can pass a 6.0 mm cuffed tracheal tube, gum-elastic bougie or fibreoptic laryngoscope through a laryngeal mask designed for intubation. A black line is present on the tube to ensure correct orientation of the mask. The sizes are 2 and $2\frac{1}{2}$ for children, 3 for adult females and 4 or 5 for adult males.

The main advantage of this technique is that the anaesthetist has both hands free to undertake other tasks. The laryngeal mask permits the measurement of the oxygen, carbon dioxide and volatile anaesthetic concentration in the expired gas.

The mask does *not* prevent gastric aspiration occurring, it is not suitable for emergency anaesthesia, and incorrect positioning can occur – which may lead to airway obstruction. This occurs in about 10% of patients, and is often due to folding back of the epiglottis as it is pushed down by the mask during insertion. An obstructed mask must be removed and repositioned.

Tracheal tube

A cuffed tracheal tube, once inserted into the trachea, maintains airway patency and minimises gastric aspiration into the lungs. All tracheal tubes have information written upon the tube (Figure 2.2).

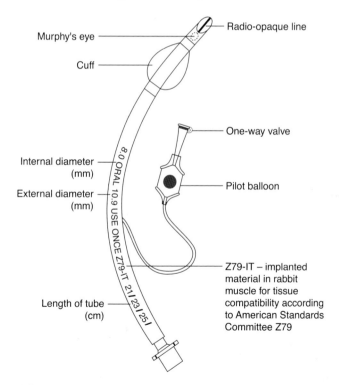

Figure 2.2 Typical tracheal tube.

The cuff is present to prevent aspiration of gastric contents. Once the tube is inserted into the trachea it is inflated with 5–10 ml of air until there is no leak of gases between the tracheal wall and the tube. Insertion of excess air into the cuff can cause it to rupture and leak. High cuff pressures can cause tracheal wall damage and mucosal ulceration.

Tracheal tubes come in many shapes and sizes. The cuff may be absent, they can be reinforced so as not to kink, they can be inserted via the oral or nasal route, and some have double lumens (for deliberately deflating one lung in thoracic surgery).

A novice anaesthetist is expected to be able to provide a detailed description of the information on a tracheal tube: it is a basic tool of the trade! The tube is inserted by holding the laryngoscope in the left hand and passing the blade into the right side of the mouth. The tongue is then pushed to the left as the blade is passed down the tongue and inserted anterior to the epiglottis in the vallecula. Elevation of the whole laryngoscope will facilitate a clear view of the glottic opening (Figure 2.3).

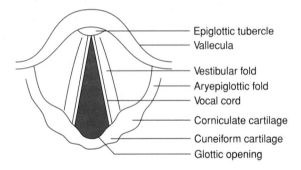

Figure 2.3 View of the larynx obtained before intubation.

Tips to aid insertion of the tracheal tube include:
- the use of a gum-elastic bougie inserted through the larynx with the tube passed over it
- the application of backwards upwards right pressure (BURP) externally over the larynx to bring it into view
- a 'helping finger' from an assistant to pull the cheek out to allow better vision in the mouth

The timely use of a gum-elastic bougie can make tracheal intubation easier and less traumatic. Occasionally, the tracheal tube impinges on the posterior rim of the larynx and will not pass smoothly over the bougie into the larynx. Rotating the tube 90° anticlockwise prevents this obstruction and facilitates intubation when using a bougie. The general principle of 'a big cannula over a small guidewire' is widely used in medicine. A size 8.0 mm tracheal tube is used for adult females and 9.0 mm for adult males. This size refers to the *internal* diameter of the tube. Tubes are normally cut to a length of 21–23 cm.

Tracheostomy

Tracheostomy can be undertaken with local anaesthesia and is used for airway control in the following circumstances:

- to bypass upper respiratory tract obstruction
- for long-term ventilation
- to facilitate suction of chest secretions
- for prevention of aspiration of gastric contents (for example, in bulbar palsy)

Percutaneous cricothyroidotomy is occasionally necessary in acute upper airway obstruction.

Nearly every general anaesthetic makes use of the facemask and Guedel airway. These simple devices are the lynchpins of safe anaesthetic airway practice. If there is any risk of aspiration of gastric contents then it is necessary to secure and protect the airway with a tracheal tube. For trainee anaesthetists we suggest that all cases needing muscle relaxation have a tracheal tube inserted. It is very easy to inadvertently ventilate the stomach with a laryngeal mask, and this can cause gastric dilatation and regurgitation of the stomach contents into the unprotected trachea. A supraglottic airway, such as the laryngeal mask, is suitable for uncomplicated cases with the patient breathing spontaneously.

2.3 Conclusion

Obstruction of the airway must be prevented at all times – a patent airway is a happy airway. Take care of the airway, and inquests will take care of themselves! (*BJA* 1925).

Chapter 3 **Tracheal intubation**

Tracheal intubation is an acquired skill. Hypoxia as a result of unrecognised oesophageal intubation can cause death. Intubation can be performed with the patient awake (local anaesthesia) or under general anaesthesia. Intubation can be achieved using the techniques shown in Box 3.1.

Box 3.1 Intubation techniques

- Above the cords
  - blind intubation
    - nasal
    - using laryngeal mask
  - larynx visualisation
    - oral ($\pm$ gum-elastic bougie)
    - laryngeal mask with fibreoptic laryngoscopy
    - fibreoptic laryngoscopy
- Below the cords
  - cricothyroid puncture
  - cricothyroidotomy
  - transtracheal ventilation
  - tracheostomy

3.1 Laryngoscopes

The laryngoscope is an important tool. It is essentially a light source on a tongue-retracting blade. Many variations exist, but it is always best to use a medium-length blade first when attempting intubation.

How to Survive in Anaesthesia: A Guide for Trainees, Fourth Edition.
Neville Robinson, George Hall and William Fawcett.
© 2012 John Wiley & Sons, Ltd. Published 2012 by John Wiley & Sons, Ltd.

The most commonly used laryngoscope, the MacIntosh laryngoscope, is a curved-blade device which allows for vision around the tongue. There must be at least two of these in every anaesthetic room. Surprisingly, the bulb often fails despite working when checked a few minutes before, so a spare laryngoscope is essential. There are many types of laryngoscopes in use, ranging from straight-bladed to video and fibreoptic models.

3.2 Laryngoscopic views

The laryngoscopic views seen on intubation are often recorded by the anaes-thetist, and have been graded by Cormack and Lehane:
- Grade I: full view of glottis
- Grade II: only posterior commissure visible
- Grade III: only tip of epiglottis visible
- Grade IV: no glottic structure visible.

3.3 Displacement

Tracheal tubes can be displaced after correct insertion. This is particularly likely when the patient is moved or the position changed. Flexion or extension of the head, or lateral neck movement, has been shown to cause movement of the tube of up to 5 cm within the trachea. Tracheal tubes should be fixed securely to minimise accidental extubation, and the correct positioning should be checked regularly.

3.4 Confirmation of tracheal intubation

Confirmation is by clinical signs and technical tests. In the operating theatre both methods are used. Elsewhere, however, only clinical signs can be used.

Clinical signs
These are listed in Box 3.2.

Box 3.2 Clinical signs used to confirm tracheal intubation

- Direct visualisation of tracheal tube through vocal cords
- Palpation of tube movement within the trachea
- Chest movements
- Breath sounds
- Reservoir bag compliance and refill
- Condensation of water vapour on clear tracheal tubes

Seeing the tracheal tube passing through the vocal cords is the best clinical method of confirming tracheal intubation. This is normally achieved easily, but is not always possible in technically difficult intubations. All anaesthetists can recount situations where they *thought* they had seen the tracheal tube pass through the vocal cords but subsequently found it in the oesophagus. The belief that the trachea is intubated can lead to a false sense of airway security if cyanosis occurs, and often other causes are sought for the hypoxaemia. The position of the tracheal tube must always be checked in these circumstances.

The other listed signs are helpful, but *unreliable*, in confirming correct placement of the tracheal tube.

Although an assistant applying cricoid pressure may 'feel' the tube passing down the trachea, the same sensation can also occur with an oesophageal intubation. Observation of chest wall movement is no guarantee of correct tracheal tube placement. It may be impossible to observe in some patients (because of obesity) and may occur also in cases of oesophageal intubation.

Auscultation can be misleading: gas movement in the oesophagus can be transmitted to the lungs, and so oesophageal sounds may be mistaken for lung sounds. Epigastric auscultation can be undertaken, but breath sounds again may be heard in the epigastrium, and so can cause confusion.

There is a characteristic 'feel' to the breathing-circuit reservoir bag, which is often different when the oesophagus is intubated. Reservoir bag refilling will occur in tracheal intubation, but has been described after stomach distension with oesophageal intubation. A 'rumbling' noise is often heard in oesophageal intubation, which is distinct from that heard in tracheal intubation.

Condensation of water vapour is more likely to be seen with tracheal intubation, but can be present in gas emanating from the stomach and so is considered unreliable. If in doubt, and if at all possible, it is worth confirming correct tracheal tube placement by viewing again the tube passing through the larynx.

Technical tests

The commonly used tests are shown in Box 3.3.

Box 3.3 Technical tests to confirm intubation

- End-tidal CO_2 monitoring – six breaths
- Fibreoptic observation of the trachea

The end-tidal CO_2 concentration can be measured using a capnograph. If pulmonary perfusion is adequate, end-tidal CO_2 concentration is about 5%.

No CO_2 is excreted from the stomach, so any CO_2 present must be from the lungs. *Six breaths of CO_2* must be seen to confirm tracheal intubation. This is because alveolar CO_2 may have been ventilated into the upper gastrointestinal tract before intubation and it will take six breaths to excrete it from the stomach. Carbonated drinks may be present occasionally in the stomach and can cause some confusion.

A fibreoptic laryngoscope placed through the tracheal tube will show if tracheal placement is correct.

Although there are many tests to confirm tracheal intubation, the 'gold standard' is six breaths of end-tidal CO_2 with visual confirmation of laryngeal placement of the tube.

3.5 Complications of tracheal intubation

The complications of intubation are shown in Box 3.4. The trainee needs to take special care to avoid the immediate complications. Tracheal tubes can easily kink or be placed too far into the trachea and either sit on the carina or pass into the right main bronchus. High airway pressures may be seen when a patient is ventilated under these circumstances. Auscultation of the chest bilaterally may reveal a different intensity of breath sounds in endobronchial intubation. The tube is then pulled back and positioned correctly. Although almost invariably the tracheal tube passes into the right main bronchus, we have managed on rare occasions to intubate the left main bronchus.

Box 3.4 Complications of tracheal intubation

- Laryngoscopy
  - trauma to mouth, teeth, pharynx and larynx
  - increased arterial pressure
  - arrhythmias
  - laryngospasm
  - bronchospasm
- Immediate
  - oesophageal placement
  - pulmonary aspiration
  - displacement of tube from trachea
  - endobronchial intubation
  - airway obstruction: tube kinked, mucous plug, tracheal cuff herniation over lower end of tube

- Long-term
  - cord ulceration with voice change
  - tracheal stenosis
  - recurrent and superior laryngeal nerve damage

3.6 Conclusion

The tracheal tube must be correctly sited and secured. Confirmation by direct observation of tracheal placement and six breaths of end-tidal CO_2 with continuous monitoring can avoid the potentially fatal consequences resulting from hypoxia. An anaesthetic maxim to remember when unsure of tracheal tube placement is:

IF IN DOUBT, TAKE IT OUT!

Patients do not die from failure to intubate but from failure to oxygenate.

Chapter 4 **Failed intubation drill**

It is essential to ask for assistance before anaesthetising patients who have been assessed as having potentially difficult airways. Failed tracheal intubation can occur in both elective and emergency anaesthesia. It is important to prepare a plan of management should intubation be impossible during the induction of general anaesthesia. We recommend that 'failed intubation drills' should be practised when juniors are accompanied by senior colleagues.

4.1 Initial strategy

The strategy for each case should be similar to that shown in Box 4.1. Calling for senior help, preventing hypoxia and not giving further doses of muscle relaxants when you are confronted by an impossible intubation are key points.

Box 4.1 Initial course of action for failed intubation

1 *Plan* a course of management before starting anaesthesia
2 Call for *HELP*
3 Maintain airway
4 Ventilate with 100% oxygen
5 Maintain cricoid pressure (if part of anaesthetic technique)
6 Avoid persistent attempts to intubate if patient is hypoxic
7 Avoid further doses of muscle relaxants until you are absolutely sure of airway control and ventilation

---

The airway must be patent and *the patient must be oxygenated*. Suxamethonium is the muscle relaxant with the fastest onset and shortest duration of

---

How to Survive in Anaesthesia: A Guide for Trainees, Fourth Edition.
Neville Robinson, George Hall and William Fawcett.
© 2012 John Wiley & Sons, Ltd. Published 2012 by John Wiley & Sons, Ltd.

action and is most commonly used for emergency surgery, in patients with full stomachs, and in those who are at risk of regurgitation (for example, hiatus hernia). Experienced anaesthetists often use muscle relaxants of slower onset for elective surgical patients in whom they can be confident of airway control. Muscle relaxants should *not* be given inappropriately, for example in cases of upper airway obstruction. If a patient is paralysed, and tracheal intubation, patency of the upper airway and oxygenation are impossible, then hypoxaemia and death will occur. Some longer-acting muscle relaxants can now be reversed quickly with a new drug called sugammadex.

Consider why intubation has failed. A common cause in emergency anaesthesia is inexpertly applied cricoid pressure. In these circumstances the larynx may need to be manipulated into view. A gum-elastic bougie is helpful for railroading tracheal tubes into position when the larynx is visible but the tube will not pass into the trachea. Do not spend time attempting these manoeuvres if the patient is becoming hypoxic.

4.2 Secondary decisions

If intubation has failed, further decisions have to be made (Box 4.2).

Box 4.2 Subsequent decisions for consideration after failed intubation

1 Awaken patient or continue anaesthetic until senior help arrives
2 Summon experienced help – intubate under general or local anaesthesia: laryngeal mask (intubation through mask), fibreoptic intubation, blind nasal intubation
3 Last resorts include retrograde intubation, transtracheal jet ventilation, cricothyroidotomy
4 Make elective tracheostomy
5 Perform surgery under regional anaesthesia

The safest decision is to awaken the patient, although this may be modified by considering the elective or emergency nature of the surgery. Patients are not usually pleased to be woken up without undergoing surgery, but at least they are alive to complain! If airway control and ventilation are easy, or the patient reverts spontaneously to breathing in an unobstructed fashion and help is nearby, the anaesthetic may be continued. A laryngeal mask can secure airway patency when other methods have failed. Sometimes it is possible to continue the anaesthetic with the patient breathing spontaneously unintubated, but intubation may be mandatory.

Intubation can be achieved through a laryngeal mask airway, by blind nasal intubation techniques or via a fibreoptic laryngoscope. Retrograde intubation can also be used occasionally. This technique involves cricothyroid membrane puncture and a guide catheter being pushed up through the larynx and out of the mouth. A tracheal tube can then be passed over the guiding catheter (the same principle as described in Chapter 3). Equipment for achieving airway control includes cricothyroid puncture devices that can be connected to a breathing circuit and transtracheal jet ventilation devices.

Formal tracheostomy may have to be considered. Abandonment of a general anaesthetic technique and implementation of surgery under regional anaesthesia is a sensible alternative.

After failed intubation, both the patient and other anaesthetists need to be informed of the difficulty in case of surgery at a later date. Therefore:
1 note grade of intubation
2 mark patient's notes boldly
3 inform patient verbally and by letter
The patient's folder containing the clinical records should be marked stating the anaesthetic problem.

4.3 Conclusion

Failed intubation should be prepared for and the priority initially should be on airway control and ventilation of the lungs. It is usually safer to awaken a patient and then consider the alternatives after consultation with a more experienced colleague.

A 'failed intubation drill' should be committed to memory very early in the training programme and be practised at regular intervals. Sooner or later it will be needed.

Remember, the objective after failed intubation is oxygenation, oxygenation, followed by **OXYGENATION.**

Chapter 5 **Vascular access**

Vascular access may be classified into venous (peripheral, central) and arterial. Even a novice anaesthetist rapidly gains expertise in peripheral venous cannulation. It is also important to become proficient in central venous cannulation and insertion of arterial cannulae, within the first few months of training. We have not included detailed practical descriptions of how to undertake these procedures; these skills are best learnt by careful instruction from a senior anaesthetist.

5.1 Peripheral venous access

With rare exceptions, and none in the case of a trainee, should a general or regional anaesthetic procedure start without intravenous access. A large-bore cannula (14 or 16 gauge) or occasionally a small cannula (21 or 23 gauge) may be used, depending on the type of surgery. Flows through peripherally placed cannulae can be surprisingly high (Table 5.1).

Table 5.1 Flow rates through typical venous cannulae

Peripheral		Central	
Gauge	Flow (ml/min)	Gauge	Flow (ml/min)
23	16		
21	21		
18·5	48		
16	121	16	110
14	251	14	230

How to Survive in Anaesthesia: A Guide for Trainees, Fourth Edition.
Neville Robinson, George Hall and William Fawcett.
© 2012 John Wiley & Sons, Ltd. Published 2012 by John Wiley & Sons, Ltd.

For any surgical procedure in which rapid blood loss may occur, nothing smaller than a 16 gauge cannula should be used. For major surgery at least one 14 gauge cannula is essential. The major determinant of the flow rate achieved through a cannula is the fourth power of the internal radius. All large-bore intravenous cannulae that are inserted before induction of anaesthesia should be placed after the intradermal infiltration of lignocaine (lidocaine) using a 25 gauge needle. The 'sting' of the local anaesthetic is trivial compared with the pain of a large intravenous cannula pushed through the skin – we speak from bitter personal experience. Be kind to your patients.

5.2 Central venous access

Central venous cannulation is undertaken to provide venous access when the peripheral route is unavailable, to measure central venous pressure, to administer drugs, and to provide parenteral nutrition.

There are two main routes by which anaesthetists acquire central venous access. First, a long venous catheter may be inserted via the basilic vein in the antecubital fossa, which will pass, one hopes, into the superior vena cava. The final position of the catheter needs confirmation by x-ray, as the catheter can pass up into the internal jugular vein and even down the other arm. There are few complications with this technique, although 'damped' pressure recordings are often seen with long catheters, and enthusiastic insertion occasionally results in the measurement of right ventricular pressures!

Second, a technique involving cannulation of the internal jugular vein is used. The internal jugular vein arises as a continuation of the sigmoid sinus as it passes through the jugular foramen. It lies within the carotid sheath, lateral to the carotid artery and the vagus nerve, and runs beneath the sternal and clavicular heads of the sternomastoid muscle, where it can be 'palpated'. It finally passes under the medial border of the clavicle to join the subclavian vein.

The right internal jugular vein is normally used, as the veins are relatively straight on the right side of the neck and the thoracic duct is avoided. The patient is placed in a head-down position to fill the veins, which avoids the risk of air embolism. A 'high-neck' approach lessens the complications, and the cannula can be inserted after ballotting the vein, or lateral to the carotid arterial pulsation. Some anaesthetists find it difficult to palpate the internal jugular vein, but it is often felt as the boggiest part of the neck lateral to the carotid artery. If the patient is hypovolaemic it can be impossible to ballotte the vein.

Central venous cannulation is now often undertaken with the assistance of ultrasound. Trainees should become proficient in the use of ultrasound early in their careers. The internal jugular vein is easy to visualise as it is compressible and lateral to the pulsating carotid artery. Strict asepsis should be used when inserting central venous cannulae. This means a surgical mask, gown and gloves and the use of a skin-cleansing agent such as chlorhexidine 2%.

Although internal jugular vein cannulation is relatively safe in skilful hands, problems can occur (Box 5.1).

Box 5.1 Complications of internal jugular vein catheterisation

- Immediate
  - venous haematoma
  - carotid artery puncture haematoma
  - pneumothorax
  - haemothorax
  - nerve trauma (brachial plexus, vagus, phrenic)
  - air embolism
- Delayed
  - infection

Haematomas are the most common, and we have been impressed by the lack of problems following inadvertent carotid artery puncture. Pneumothorax should not occur with the 'high-neck' approach. If you have more than 4 cm of the needle inserted and still have not found the vein, stop and try a different site.

Central venous pressure is measured from the midaxillary line via a pressure transducer. There is no normal central venous pressure. It is the response to an intravenous fluid load that determines whether the patient is hypovolaemic or not. The causes of variants in central venous pressure are shown in Box 5.2.

Box 5.2 Variants in central venous pressure

- Low pressure
  - hypovolaemia
  - respiratory phase variation
- High pressure
  - hypervolaemia
  - right ventricular dysfunction
  - increased right ventricular afterload

- pulmonary hypertension
- parenchymal pulmonary disease
- pneumothorax
- haemothorax
- left heart failure
- atrial arrhythmias
- tricuspid valve disease

5.3 Arterial access

This is commonly performed via the radial artery with a 20 or 22 gauge cannula. An Allen's test may be done to assess the relative contributions of the radial and ulnar arteries to blood flow of the hand. This is done by occluding both the radial and ulnar arteries and then watching for 'palmar flushing' when the ulnar artery is released. If flushing occurs, then it implies that, in the event of radial artery trauma or occlusion, the ulnar artery will supply the hand. In practice, we never bother with Allen's test as its value is not proven. Complications of arterial cannulation include thrombosis, infection, fistula, aneurysm and distal ischaemia. These are rare but, in the event of clinical ischaemia, the cannula should be removed and expert help sought urgently. Colour-coding of arterial cannulae and their dedicated infusion tubing with red tags and red three-way taps should be undertaken if possible. This reduces the risk of inadvertent injection of drugs into arteries. We have seen the results of such accidents – gangrenous fingers are most unpleasant.

5.4 Conclusion

Intravenous access is mandatory before starting any form of anaesthesia, local or general. If there is *any* possibility of rapid blood loss, insert a large-bore intravenous cannula. Lack of vascular access is a major contributor to anaesthetic disasters.

Chapter 6 **Intravenous fluids**

Intravenous fluids and electrolytes are administered, often empirically, to re-place or maintain the body's requirements. Patients are starved preoperatively to ensure an empty stomach. There is much debate on how long a patient should be without fluids or food before elective surgery: 6 hours is often taken as the minimum requirement for food and 2 hours for clear fluids, but many patients starve overnight for at least 12 hours before anaesthesia.

Once you have inserted an intravenous cannula, it is necessary to give an appropriate fluid. The main choice is between crystalloid or colloid solutions. There are also glucose-containing solutions, but it is difficult to make a case for the continued use of such solutions. There is considerable debate on the relative merits of crystalloid or colloid solutions. In practice, most anaesthetists start with 1–2 litres of crystalloid and follow this with a similar volume of colloid solution in major surgery.

Fluids are given intraoperatively to:
- replace existing deficits
- maintain fluid balance
- replace surgical loss

The existing fluid deficit can be high, particularly in bowel surgery where enemas are used and with prolonged starvation in a warm environment; 1 litre of crystalloid given intravenously at the start of anaesthesia often only replaces an existing deficit.

The rate of fluid replacement is determined by assessing the adequacy of the circulating blood volume using the following indices:
- arterial pressure
- heart rate
- central venous pressure (if available)

How to Survive in Anaesthesia: A Guide for Trainees, Fourth Edition.
Neville Robinson, George Hall and William Fawcett.
© 2012 John Wiley & Sons, Ltd. Published 2012 by John Wiley & Sons, Ltd.

- urine output
- peripheral temperature (if available)

The composition of commonly used intravenous fluids is shown in Table 6.1.

Table 6.1 Electrolytic composition of intravenous solutions (mmol/l)

Solution	Na	K	Ca	Cl	Lactate
0.9% Sodium chloride	154	–	–	154	–
Hartmann's solution	131	5	2	111	29
5% Glucose	–	–	–	–	–
4% Glucose in 0.18% NaCl	30	–	–	30	–
Haemaccel	145	5	6	145	–
Volplex	154	–	–	125	–
Gelofusine	154	–	–	120	–
Hydroxyethyl starch	154	–	–	154	–

6.1 Crystalloids

Crystalloids are isotonic solutions that have a similar fluid and electrolyte composition to the extracellular fluid. These solutions are confined to the extracellular space in a ratio of 1:3 in terms of intravascular:interstitial volume. The two commonly available solutions are Hartmann's solution and 0.9% sodium chloride solution. The lactate in Hartmann's solution is either oxidised in the liver, or undergoes gluconeogenesis. Both metabolic pathways use hydrogen ions, so mild alkalinisation occurs. It is important to remember that both these solutions add little to the intravascular volume. It has been suggested that 0.9% sodium chloride should be avoided because of the risk of hyperchloraemic acidosis. Clinically this is very rare. Normal maintenance requirements for adult patients are about 50–100 mmol/day of sodium, 40–80 mmol/day of potassium and 2–3 litres/day of water.

6.2 Glucose-containing solutions

It is difficult to make a case for continuing the use of these solutions. The stress of surgery increases circulating blood glucose, so the addition of more glucose intravenously exacerbates the metabolic insult. Furthermore, when glucose is eventually oxidised to water and carbon dioxide, the infusion is then equivalent to water (5% glucose) or a very weak hypotonic solution (4% glucose + 0.18% sodium chloride). The main reason for continuing to use these solutions seems to be the fear of the phase of sodium retention that inevitably accompanies surgery. Since low plasma sodium concentrations are almost invariably found postoperatively, this fear is unsubstantiated – patients usually need more sodium. Only a small proportion of glucose-containing solutions stay within the intravascular space; they are of little value in maintaining the blood volume.

6.3 Colloids

These are large molecules suspended in solution. They generate a colloid osmotic pressure and are confined to the intravascular space. They rarely cause allergic reactions as a side effect. Elimination is via the kidneys. There are two main types in clinical practice:
- modified gelatins
- hydroxyethyl starch

The modified gelatins are Haemaccel (polygeline), Volplex (succinylated gelatin) and Gelofusine (succinylated gelatin). The electrolytic composition and properties are shown in Tables 6.1 and 6.2, respectively, the properties being compared with those of albumin. Haemaccel contains calcium, which can cause clotting in an intravenous infusion set when it becomes mixed with citrated blood and plasma.

Table 6.2 Properties of colloid solutions

	MW	Plasma $t_{1/2}$ (h)	Elimination	Anaphylaxis
Albumin	69,000	24	Slow	Nil
Haemaccel	30,000	3	Rapid	Rare
Gelofusine	30,000	3	Rapid	Rare
Hetastarch 6%	450,000	24	Slow	Rare
Pentastarch 6–10%	200,000	2.5	Rapid	Rare
Tetrastarch 6%	130,000	2	Rapid	Rare

Hydroxyethyl starch is taken up by the reticuloendothelial system after phagocytosis in the blood, and this results in its prolonged degradation and elimination. The maximum dose is limited to 20 ml/kg/day for 10% starch solutions and 30–50 ml/kg/day for 6% starch solutions.

6.4 Conclusion

Fluid therapy is simple. Start with 1–2 litres crystalloid solution (Hartmann's solution) and follow this, if necessary, with a suitable colloid solution. This regimen has stood the test of time. Do not use glucose-containing solutions without a good reason and, if there is marked blood loss, consider red cell replacement (see Chapter 12).

Chapter 7 **The anaesthetic machine**

The anaesthetic machine delivers known gas and vapour concentrations, which are variable in amount and composition. The machine is of a 'continuous-flow' nature and designed so that gases are delivered at safe pressures. Know your machine and you will be a safe anaesthetist.

The machine has six basic components (Box 7.1).

Box 7.1 Anaesthetic machine components

- Gas supply – cylinders, pipelines and pressure gauges
- Pressure regulators
- Flowmeter needle valves
- Rotameters – or electronic readout
- Vaporisers
- Common gas outlet

Anaesthetic machines vary in age, and the different nomenclature for pressure readings can cause confusion. The derived SI (Système Internationale) unit of pressure is the pascal (Pa), and pressure in the anaesthetic machine is measured in kilopascals (kPa). The comparative factors for other units of pressure are shown in Box 7.2.

Box 7.2 One atmosphere of pressure (various units)

- 760 mm Hg
- 1034 cm H_2O

How to Survive in Anaesthesia: A Guide for Trainees, Fourth Edition.
Neville Robinson, George Hall and William Fawcett.
© 2012 John Wiley & Sons, Ltd. Published 2012 by John Wiley & Sons, Ltd.

- 15 lb/in^2
- 101 kPa
- 1 bar

7.1 Gas supply

Cylinders

These are made of molybdenum steel and are colour-coded:
- N_2O: blue body, blue shoulder
- O_2:   black body, white shoulder
- Air: grey body, white/black shoulder
- CO_2:   grey body, grey shoulder

To prevent incorrect placement of the cylinder onto the machine, a pin-index system has been devised. On each cylinder is an arrangement of three holes specific to the gas, and there is a corresponding pin on the machine. A washer (Bodok seal) is necessary on the top pin to stop leaks occurring between the cylinder and the machine. Carbon dioxide cylinders should not be connected routinely to the anaesthetic machine for fear of inadvertent use. Newer machines cannot deliver carbon dioxide.

An oxygen cylinder contains gas, and the pressure in a full cylinder is 137×100 kPa. The pressure decreases linearly as the cylinder empties. Nitrous oxide is a liquefied gas at a pressure of 52×100 kPa. The pressure in the cylinder remains the same as it empties, until all the liquid becomes gaseous (when the cylinder is about a quarter full) and then the pressure drops quite rapidly.

Pipelines

Pipelines from a central supply can be connected directly to the machine. These are again colour-coded:
- O_2:   white
- N_2O: blue
- suction pipeline: yellow

They are made of copper, and outlets from the pipeline system are identified by name, colour and shape. They have non-interchangeable Schrader valve connections.

Oxygen normally comes from a liquid cryogenic source, and nitrous oxide from central banks of cylinders. The pressure of pipeline-supplied gases is 4×100 kPa.

Pressure regulators

Beneath the machine are pressure-reducing valves which regulate the pressure entering the machine (Figure 7.1). Gas at high pressure enters and passes through a small port to a low-pressure chamber. As the pressure here rises, the diaphragm is pushed up against the spring and the valve is closed. If the outlet valve is opened, the pressure drops and the spring will push the diaphragm down, and the whole process starts again. Pressure of all gases now entering the machine is 4×100 kPa.

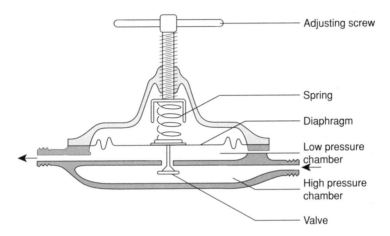

Figure 7.1 A pressure-reducing valve.

Flowmeter needle valve

The pressure is about atmospheric at the common gas outlet of the machine, and the main pressure drop from 4×100 kPa occurs across the needle valve at the base of the rotameters.

The knobs are colour-coded; in addition, the oxygen knob is bigger than the others and of a wider, grooved nature. This enables it to be identified in darkness. In the United Kingdom it is the convention for the oxygen valve to be mounted on the left side of the machine.

Rotameters

These are calibrated specifically for each gas and are non-interchangeable. Cracks in the rotameter tubing may lead to hypoxic mixtures being produced, so an oxygen gas analyser is positioned at the common gas outlet on the machine.

The scale on the rotameter is often non-linear, as the rotameters themselves are tapered. Low gas flows, when using carbon dioxide absorption circuits, need to be very accurate. Newer machines have a digital readout of the delivery of gases and do not use rotameters.

Vaporisers

These convert a volatile liquid anaesthetic to a continuous-flow anaesthetic vapour mixed with gases, under controlled conditions. Thermal energy is used in converting a liquid to a vapour, and a temperature drop occurs within the liquid. Variable rates of vaporisation will occur unless this is compensated for. Temperature compensation (Tec-type) vaporisers are in common use, and compensation is achieved by means of a bimetallic strip within the machine.

A vaporiser should be constructed of materials of high specific heat and high thermal conductivity. Within the vaporiser are a series of copper helical wicks which provide a large surface area, ensuring that a saturated vapour pressure exists within the vaporiser at all times.

Vaporisers should be filled at the end of the operating list to decrease pollution. There is a non-interchangeable filling device that ensures that the vaporiser is filled with the correct agent. Vaporisers are connected to the 'back bar' of the anaesthetic machine and an O-ring washer system must be present at this site to stop leaks.

Common gas outlet

The gases finally pass from the machine via the common gas outlet at about atmospheric pressure. The oxygen analyser is connected here.

In addition to the Bourdon-type pressure gauges, which measure the cylinder and pipeline pressure, three other features on the machine must be noted:

- *Oxygen flush.* This button delivers oxygen at a rate of 30 litres/minute to the common gas outlet, bypassing the vaporisers and flowmeters.
- *Hypoxic or oxygen failure alarm.* This device causes the nitrous oxide to be cut or dumped if the oxygen supply is < 21%. This can occur if the oxygen rotameter is accidentally bumped or turned down, or if it fails electronically. An audible alarm is heard when this is activated.
- *Pressure relief valve.* On the 'back bar' between the common gas outlet and the vaporisers, there is a pressure release valve which protects the machine against excessive pressure caused by obstruction to gas flow beyond the common gas outlet. This does not protect the patient but is designed to protect the machine. It is activated by back pressure in excess of a third of an atmosphere (35 kPa).

7.2 Checking the anaesthetic machine

Absolute familiarity with the anaesthetic machine is fundamental for safe practice. It *must* be checked before an operating list, and 10 items need inspection (Box 7.3). These checks are the responsibility of the anaesthetist. A checklist is normally attached to the anaesthetic machine.

Box 7.3 Anaesthetic machine checklist

- Anaesthetic machine
- Monitoring devices
- Gas supply
  - tug test
  - flowmeters
- Vaporisers
- Breathing systems
- Ventilator
- Scavenging system
- Ancillary equipment – particularly suction
- Alternative means of ventilating patient
- Recording

Anaesthetic machine

Check that the machine and ancillary equipment are connected to the electrical supply and switched on. Note should be taken of any information attached to the machine. Special attention should be taken after routine maintenance by service engineers when 'first user notices' are fixed prominently to the anaesthetic machine. Some newer machines perform a self-test.

Monitoring devices

Check that these devices (especially the oxygen analyser, pulse oximeter and capnograph) are functioning and have appropriate alarm limits. Sampling lines should be unobstructed and an appropriate frequency of non-invasive blood pressure measurement selected. The oxygen analyser is a fuel cell which is normally calibrated by a single-point calibration to room air – 21%. The sensor should be attached firmly to the common gas outlet.

Gas supply

This is done to ensure that the correct gas supplies and connections exist within the machine, to check pressures and to stop the accidental delivery of a hypoxic gas mixture. These checks, with familiarity, take about 5 minutes:

- Note the gases supplied by pipelines and confirm that each pipeline is appropriately inserted into its gas supply terminal by undertaking a 'tug test'.
- Check that there is an oxygen supply and that a reserve oxygen cylinder is available.
- Check that the other gases available are connected securely, seated and turned off after checking their contents. Carbon dioxide cylinders should not be present on the anaesthetic machine. Ensure that blanking plugs are fitted onto empty cylinder yokes. A full oxygen cylinder has a pressure of 137×100 kPa and a nitrous oxide cylinder has a pressure of 52×100 kPa until only a quarter full.
- All pipeline pressure gauges should indicate 4×100 kPa.
- Check that the flowmeter works smoothly and that the bobbins, if present, move freely without sticking. Check that the anti-hypoxia device is working correctly.
- Check the emergency oxygen bypass control function.

Vaporisers
- Check that the vaporiser is adequately filled.
- Check O-rings present on back bar.
- Check for correct mounting and filling, and that the back bar is locked.
- Turn 'on' – check for leaks – turn 'off' – recheck for leaks (check for leaks by occluding common gas outlet after opening oxygen rotameter).
- Turn off vaporisers.
- Repeat test immediately after changing any vaporiser.

Breathing systems
- A new single-use bacterial/viral filter and catheter mount must be used for each patient.
- Check the configuration of the system.
- Check for leaks in the reservoir bag and that the adjustable, pressure-limiting expiratory valve does not stick and can be fully opened and closed.
- Check for leaks in the circuit.
- Check tightness of all connections (push-and-twist technique).
- Check the unidirectional valves in a circular system and in the exhaust system.
- Check for patency and flow of gas through the whole system.

Ventilator
- Check that it is configured appropriately for its intended use.
- Check for familiarity with the ventilator.

- Check tubing security and configuration.
- Check that the pressure relief valve functions at the correct pressure.
- Check that the alarm system works and set alarm limits.
- Set controls and ensure that an adequate pressure is generated during the inspiratory phase.

Scavenging system
- Check that it is switched on and functioning correctly and that the tubing is attached to the appropriate exhaust point of the breathing system or ventilator.

Ancillary equipment
- Check that all laryngoscopes, intubation aids, forceps, bougies etc. are present and working. Appropriately sized face masks, airways, tracheal tubes and connectors must be checked (including patency).
- Check that the suction is working and connections are secure.
- Check that the patient trolley, bed or table can be tilted head-down rapidly.

Alternative means of ventilating patient
- Check that a self-inflating bag and filled oxygen cylinder are in close proximity (alternative means of ventilating patient if there is a ventilator failure).

Recording
- Sign and date the logbook kept with the anaesthetic machine (confirm machine checked).
- Record on each patient's anaesthetic chart that the anaesthetic machine, breathing system and monitoring have been checked.

7.3 Conclusion

The novice anaesthetist must have a thorough knowledge of the basic workings of an anaesthetic machine, and checking the machine must become a regular habit. The start of work in operating theatres should be signalled by a cacophony of alarms, as all the machines are checked before use.

Do not assume, however, that, because the machine was checked early in the morning, nothing can go wrong for the rest of the day. Machines are moved and knocked, pipelines are stretched and vaporisers are changed. **Remain vigilant.**

Chapter 8 **Anaesthetic breathing systems**

Anaesthetic breathing systems are classified into three main groups:
- systems using carbon dioxide absorption
- rebreathing systems
- non-rebreathing systems

8.1 Components

Each circuit consists of a variable number of components and is often made as a single unit, rather than needing to be assembled from individual items (Box 8.1).

Box 8.1 Anaesthetic breathing circuit components

- Breathing hoses
- Bags
- Adjustable pressure-limiting valves (APL)
- Connections
- Carbon dioxide absorption
- Unidirectional valves

Breathing hoses
These are corrugated, 22 mm diameter, plastic tubes which are non-kinkable and non-compliant. They have a volume of 400–450 ml/m, and the newer plastic hoses are more prone to pin-hole leaks than older rubber hoses, so circuits must be checked.

How to Survive in Anaesthesia: A Guide for Trainees, Fourth Edition.
Neville Robinson, George Hall and William Fawcett.
© 2012 John Wiley & Sons, Ltd. Published 2012 by John Wiley & Sons, Ltd.

Bags

These are made of rubber and are of 2 litre volume in adult circuits and 500 ml volume in paediatric circuits. They have four functions (Box 8.2).

Box 8.2 Functions of bags in breathing systems

- Reservoir for gases. Although the machine can deliver flow rates of up to 10–20 litres/min of gas, the patient has brief inspiratory flow rates of up to 30 litres/min. To facilitate the delivery of this high flow rate, there must be a reservoir.
- Monitoring of ventilation.
- Facilitating manual intermittent positive pressure ventilation.
- Pressure-limiting function. The bag can distend to large volumes without pressure within the system increasing greatly. This safety feature avoids barotrauma to the patient's lungs if the pressure-limiting valve malfunctions or is omitted from the circuit.

Adjustable pressure-limiting valves (APL)

These variable-orifice, variable-resistance devices vent excess gases. They often have a scavenging facility. They consist of a light disc held onto a circular knife-edge by a light spring with tension. The spring is adjusted by a screw thread.

When the valve is set fully open, the pressure to open the disc, and hence the valve, is only 0.1–0.2 kPa (1–2 cm H_2O), and minimal resistance to flow occurs. When the valve is closed, a safety device protects the patient by opening at a pressure of about 6 kPa (60 cm H_2O). This occurs at a gas flow of 30 litres/minute.

Connections

Connections are achieved by 22 mm or 15 mm male-to-female fittings.

Carbon dioxide absorption

Sodalime is used for this. It contains 80% calcium hydroxide, 4% sodium hydroxide, 1% potassium hydroxide and the remainder is water. It contains an indicator, which changes colour as the mixture is exhausted, and a hardener – silica gel. It is easy to underestimate how much sodalime is 'exhausted' when checking the anaesthetic machine. It is sensible to ensure that there is enough fresh sodalime available for the whole operating session, as it is difficult to replace it in the middle of an operation.

Absorption occurs via the following chemical reaction:

$$CO_2 + H_2O \rightarrow H_2CO_3$$

$$H_2CO_3 + 2NaOH \rightarrow Na_2CO_3 + 2H_2O$$

$$Na_2CO_3 + Ca(OH)_2 \rightarrow CaCO_3 + 2NaOH$$

Potassium hydroxide behaves similarly to sodium hydroxide. Heat is produced in this reaction. Small amounts of gases and vapours are also absorbed.

Unidirectional valves

These ensure one-way flow in circle systems.

8.2 Systems using carbon dioxide absorption

The circle system has unidirectional valves to direct gas flow through hoses, a reservoir bag, and sodalime. Oxygen and the volatile vapour are added. As the inspired gases are free of carbon dioxide, the patient can rebreathe without adverse physiological effects. Low gas flows can be used, and the rotameters, or digital readouts, must be accurate.

The system is economical, conserves heat and moisture, and decreases pollution. However, to be efficient it must be free from leaks. Oxygen, carbon dioxide and anaesthetic vapour analysis is mandatory. Dilution of gases in the reservoir bag by nitrogen in the early part of the anaesthetic can occur – higher gas flows in the first 5 minutes are recommended.

Oxygen uptake from the lungs is relatively constant at 200–250 ml/min, but nitrous oxide uptake is high initially (500 ml/min), falling to 200 ml/min after 30 minutes, and 100 ml/min after 60 minutes. Therefore, hypoxic mixtures are possible at low flows – and this is one reason why an oxygen analyser must be incorporated into the system. The use of very low fresh gas flows with the circle system can lead to an increased risk of awareness at the start of surgery if volatile agents are used. Flow rates greater than 3 litres/minute minimise this problem.

The position of the vaporiser in the circuit is important. It is usually outside the circle (VOC) when conventional vaporisers can be used.

8.3 Rebreathing systems

Traditionally these systems have no separation of the inspired and expired gases, although in the newer coaxial systems partition of the gases occurs. Under conditions of low fresh gas flow or hyperventilation of the patient, rebreathing of carbon dioxide is possible. Flow rates of gases should be adjusted according to capnography. Classification of rebreathing systems was first described by Mapleson in 1954. There are six basic systems (Figure 8.1) and two involving a coaxial arrangement (Figure 8.2).

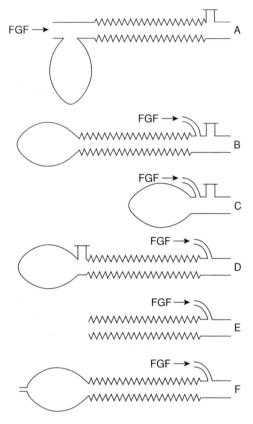

Figure 8.1 Mapleson classification of rebreathing systems. Arrows indicate direction of fresh gas flow (FGF).

The *Mapleson A* is also called the Magill attachment. Fresh gas flow should equal alveolar minute ventilation for spontaneous respiration and be 2–2.5 times the alveolar minute ventilation for intermittent positive pressure ventilation. This is the most efficient system for spontaneously breathing patients and the least efficient for intermittent positive pressure ventilation. The system is heavy with the valve in its traditional position and access is often difficult; because of this it was modified by Lack to incorporate the valve at

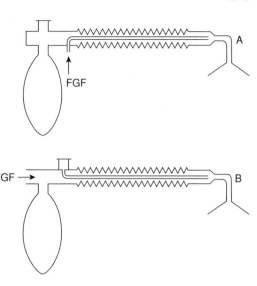

Figure 8.2 Coaxial systems of (A) Bain and (B) Lack. FGF, fresh gas flow.

the machine end of the circuit by an external tubing modification (parallel Lack circuit).

The *Mapleson B* and *C* systems are used infrequently, but the C is useful for brief periods of manual ventilation.

The *Mapleson D, E* and *F* systems are T-pieces at the patient end of the circuit and differ only in the way they vent the gases. The Mapleson D is the most efficient for intermittent positive pressure ventilation.

The *Bain* circuit is a coaxial Mapleson D with a 22 mm diameter outer tube and a 7 mm diameter inner tube. The gases enter via the inner tube. It is light, often disposable, has the gas entry and the expiratory valve at the machine end, and has a clear outer tube to ensure that the inner tube can be seen to be attached and not kinked. Leaks or holes in the inner tubing cause rapid carbon dioxide rebreathing. To check that there are no leaks in the inner tube, it should be occluded (fifth finger or 2 ml syringe). Oxygen flows of 5 litres/min into the system will cause the anaesthetic machine back-bar pressure-releasing alarm to blow as the occlusion pressure is transmitted along the machine. The reservoir bag should *not* distend.

Flow rates using this system are high; at least 70–100 ml/kg/min and up to 2–3 times the minute alveolar ventilation are recommended, but this can be adjusted according to capnography.

The *Mapleson E* and *F* systems incorporate the Ayre's T-piece, have no adjustable pressure limiting valves, and are used for children under 20–25 kg, again at flows of 2–3 times the minute alveolar ventilation. The open-ended reservoir bag of the Jackson–Rees modification (Mapleson F) was added to assist intermittent positive pressure ventilation rather than occluding the end of the Mapleson E system, although spontaneous ventilation can be monitored by its movement.

8.4 Non-rebreathing systems

These use one-way, or non-rebreathing, valves to direct and separate the inspired and expired gases. They are not used in the operating theatre, but are seen in the 'draw-over' system for field anaesthesia where compressed gases are unavailable (Triservice devices). They are low-resistance systems, as the patient's inspiratory efforts cause gas flow, and a low-resistance draw-over vaporiser must be used. Inflating bellows can be added for ventilation purposes.

8.5 Conclusion

Anaesthetic breathing circuits may appear confusing initially, but the principles are simple. Modern monitoring facilities, particularly capnography and oxygen analysis, enable appropriate fresh gas flows to be used whatever circuit is employed. The breathing circuits are the most common site for gas leaks. **Check carefully.**

Chapter 9 **Ventilators and other equipment**

9.1 Ventilators

Ventilation can be delivered to the lung by two methods.

- *Negative pressure devices.* A negative pressure is applied externally around the thorax (cuirass ventilators).
- *Positive pressure devices.* A positive pressure is applied to the lungs via the trachea. This is the method used in theatre, and these devices are driven by one of three methods: gas, electricity, or a separate supply of compressed air or oxygen.

There are five types of ventilators (Box 9.1).

Box 9.1 Types of ventilators

- Mechanical thumbs
- Minute volume dividers
- Bag squeezers
- Intermittent flow generators
- High-frequency ventilators

Mechanical thumbs are used only with T-piece circuits. Bag squeezers are widely used with circle systems where a pneumatic bellows device operates intermittently.

Intermittent flow generators have a control mechanism that intermittently interrupts a flow of gas from a high-pressure source (for example, a cylinder). These can be made compact and are used for ventilation during transportation. High-frequency ventilators deliver very small tidal volumes at very high rates to maintain normal gas exchange.

How to Survive in Anaesthesia: A Guide for Trainees, Fourth Edition.
Neville Robinson, George Hall and William Fawcett.
© 2012 John Wiley & Sons, Ltd. Published 2012 by John Wiley & Sons, Ltd.

A typical example of a minute volume divider is the Manley ventilator, still sometimes found in an anaesthetic room.

Flow-generated ventilators are now commonly used in the operating theatres and intensive care units and deliver a fixed total volume irrespective of alterations in lung compliance. Ventilators now have a *hypoxic guard*, which means that it is impossible to deliver a mixture of gases that has a concentration of less than 25% oxygen. Newer ventilators are sophisticated. They perform a self-check. Gases can be delivered to a set tidal volume or pressure, PEEP (positive end-expiratory pressures) can be applied to the patient's lungs, inspiration/expiration ratios can be altered. For nearly all routine anaesthesia these complexities can be ignored.

Never use a ventilator unless you have received clear instructions about how it functions. Most patients anaesthetised in theatre require only simple ventilators, and the trend towards increasing complexity is to be deplored. We have seen recently a ventilator that had over 30 possible settings. Although it may be of value in intensive care, in theatre it is a disaster waiting to happen. The ideal ventilator has no more than three knobs!

You must ensure that the following are set appropriately when using a ventilator:
- the correct mode of ventilation (usually controlled mandatory ventilation, CMV)
- tidal volume (e.g. 8 ml/kg)
- breaths/minute (e.g. 10–12)
- inspiratory/expiratory (I/E) ratio (often 1 : 2)
- pressure limit (usually < 30 mm Hg)
- positive end-expiratory pressure (PEEP) of 0–4 mm Hg
- alarm settings are on and correct

Whenever the lungs are ventilated it is *imperative* that the following monitoring is available:
- disconnection alarm
- expired minute volume
- capnography
- inspired oxygen concentration beyond the ventilator
- airway pressure

Other monitoring may be used, as required. However, the basic monitoring ensures that the circuit is intact without leaks and that ventilation is adequate with a suitable inspired oxygen concentration. If in doubt, check that the lungs are being ventilated by observation and auscultation.

9.2 Suction devices

These consist of three basic components (Box 9.2).

Box 9.2 Suction device components

- *Vacuum generating pump.* This is normally located centrally within the hospital. The yellow piping in theatre is non-interchangeable and the suction system is connected to a high-volume displacement pump that is linked by a series of anticontamination traps to a central reservoir.
- *Reservoir* in theatre to contain the fluid aspirated. A filter with a float mechanism exists within the reservoir to stop contamination of the pump by aspirated fluid.
- *Delivery tubing,* which is disposable and is connected to flexible or rigid (Yankauer) catheters. Prolonged tracheal suction can cause lung collapse and bradycardia, and should not be used.

The acceptable flow rate for suction devices is 35 litres/minute of air at a maximum of 80 kPa negative pressure.

9.3 Scavenging apparatus

Chronic and short-term exposure to inhalational anaesthetic agents is considered to be detrimental to the health of theatre workers, although there is no conclusive evidence of impaired concentration, physical health, or fetal well-being in pregnant women.

On balance it seems sensible to scavenge waste gases. Scavenging systems consist of three components (Box 9.3).

Box 9.3 Scavenging system components

- *Collecting system.* This is a shroud enclosing the APL valve of the breathing system. The connection is of 30 mm diameter to prevent accidental connection to the breathing system circuit (22 mm).
- *Receiving system.* This has a reservoir to ensure adequate removal of gases. A rubber bag, or a rigid bottle, is often used, and this ensures that removal of gases occurs even if the volume cleared is less than the peak expiratory flow rate.

- *Disposal system.* Three systems are used to remove the gases:
  - passive, through wide-bore tubing to a terminal ventilator in the roof: disposal is dependent on wind direction.
  - assisted passive: the air-conditioning system extractor ducts remove the gases.
  - active: a dedicated ejector flowmeter or fan system is used. A low-pressure, high-volume system able to remove 75 l/min (with a peak flow of 130 l/min) is used.

9.4 Humidification

Humidification of inspired air occurs in the nose and naso/oropharynx. It is saturated by the time it reaches the trachea. Delivery of dry gases to the trachea by tracheal tubes can cause decreased ciliary activity, tenacious mucus and even atelectasis.

In the operating theatre, humidification is usually carried out by a passive method using a 'heat and moisture exchanger' filter. The filter is connected between the breathing circuit and the laryngeal mask or tracheal tube. A hydrophobic membrane within the filter acts to retain water vapour and heat, and helps maintain the humidity of the anaesthetic gases in the patient's respiratory tract. The filter is disposable, has a low resistance to gas flow and removes bacteria and viruses. It prevents contamination of the breathing circuit and must be changed after every patient.

9.5 Conclusion

Ventilators should never be used unless you have received clear instructions about their function.

Beware of disconnections and ensure appropriate monitoring is in place. Suction apparatus must be checked and available wherever anaesthesia is undertaken.

Make sure that you are not the only sucker in theatre!

Chapter 10 **Monitoring in anaesthesia**

An important source of anaesthetic-related morbidity and mortality remains human error. All anaesthetists have tales of drug administration errors and 'near-misses'; those anaesthetists who claim never to have problems are either doing insufficient work or are economical with the truth. A critical incident register is recommended in every anaesthetic department. A critical incident is an untoward event, which, if left uncorrected, would have led to anaesthetic-related mortality or morbidity. It includes many events ranging from disconnection of the breathing circuit to unrecognised oesophageal intubation and severe bronchospasm. It is hoped that better monitoring will reduce the incidence of these complications.

There should be appropriate monitoring wherever anaesthesia is conducted, whether it is in the anaesthetic room, the operating theatre, the psychiatric department, the x-ray department, or a dental surgery.

Indeed, anaesthetising 'away from home' outside the operating theatres demands particular care, and appropriate monitoring *must be present*.

Monitoring facilities have improved greatly in recent years but still fall short of two essential requirements:
• the ability to monitor cerebral oxygenation;
• the ability to monitor accurately the depth of anaesthesia (many false dawns). Full monitoring has three requirements, as shown in Box 10.1.

Box 10.1 Anaesthesia monitoring requirements

• Presence of anaesthetist
• Checking and monitoring the anaesthetic equipment
• Patient monitoring
  − clinical
  − technical

How to Survive in Anaesthesia: A Guide for Trainees, Fourth Edition.
Neville Robinson, George Hall and William Fawcett.
© 2012 John Wiley & Sons, Ltd. Published 2012 by John Wiley & Sons, Ltd.

10.1 Anaesthetist

The anaesthetist *must* be present throughout the whole surgical procedure, and must be readily available to recovery room staff until the patient leaves the theatre complex. *This responsibility is solely the anaesthetist's*, and is applicable in general and regional anaesthesia, and also in some sedation techniques where the anaesthetist is involved.

An adequate record must be made of the whole anaesthetic process, from the induction to full recovery of the patient. Errors can occur for a variety of reasons, ranging from inexperience and lack of training to tiredness, boredom and inattention. Vigilance in an anaesthetist is a function of self-motivation.

The novice anaesthetist should acquire rigorous monitoring habits. Tracheal intubation must be confirmed *every* time, and the equipment, the anaesthetic machine and circuitry checked as a routine. Postoperative visits to assess a patient's progress are salutary and give an opportunity to improve aspects of care, including postoperative analgesia and the prevention of nausea and vomiting.

10.2 Checking and monitoring equipment

Checking and monitoring the function of anaesthetic equipment has already been discussed in preceding chapters. Two key features must be emphasised – the oxygen supply and the breathing system.

Oxygen supply

The gas supply to the oxygen flowmeter must contain a low-pressure warning device and have an audible alarm.

If hypoxic mixtures can be delivered (most old machines), then a device which continuously monitors the concentration of oxygen delivered to the patient must be fitted, and this too must have an audible alarm.

Breathing system

If faults exist in the circuit, these are best detected by monitoring the expired volume and the end-tidal carbon dioxide concentration and by measuring the airway pressure (high-pressure alarm). Clinical observation of the reservoir bag may reveal leaks, disconnections and overdistension from high pressure. During mechanical ventilation measurement of the airway pressure, the expired volume, and the oxygen and carbon dioxide concentrations is mandatory (see Chapter 9).

The alarm limits for equipment should be reset for each case, and alarms should be turned ON (not turned off because the limits are being exceeded for a particular patient, but are not causing concern).

10.3 Patient monitoring

Clinical

The continuous observation of the patient's colour, chest movement and pattern of respiration, absence or presence of sweating and lacrimation, re-actions of the pupil, palpation of a peripheral pulse and use of a stethoscope provide essential basic monitoring of the patient. Much useful information can be obtained by simple observation, palpation and auscultation – arts that are rapidly disappearing from anaesthesia.

Technical

The circulation and ventilation need continuous monitoring in all forms of anaesthesia. If muscle relaxants are used, a peripheral nerve stimulator should be used. The devices used routinely are shown in Box 10.2.

Box 10.2 Patient monitoring devices (essential)

- Cardiovascular
  - heart rate
  - electrocardiogram
  - non-invasive arterial pressure
  - oximeter
- Respiratory
  - respiratory rate
  - end-tidal carbon dioxide concentration
  - inspired oxygen
- Muscle relaxation
  - peripheral nerve stimulator
- Gas analysis and minimum alveolar concentration (MAC)

In specialised surgery, facilities for further monitoring are required (Box 10.3).

Box 10.3 Specialised patient monitoring devices

- Invasive arterial pressure
- Central venous pressure
- Pulmonary artery pressure
- Cardiac output (oesophageal Doppler)
- Urine output

- Temperature measurement
- Measurement of blood loss
- Biochemical analysis: pH, arterial gas analysis, electrolytes
- Haematological analysis: haemoglobin, coagulation studies

The *electrocardiogram* needs special emphasis because it is important to remember that electrical activity can exist even though there is no adequate cardiac output. Its value lies principally in monitoring changes in heart rate and in the diagnosis of arrhythmias. ST segment changes can also be noted.

Oximetry depends upon the differing absorption of light at different wavelengths by the various states of haemoglobin. Oxyhaemoglobin and reduced haemoglobin differ at both the red and infrared portions of the spectrum. The absorption is the same at 805 nm, the isobestic point. A pulse oximeter has two light sources on one side of the probe and a photodiode which generates a voltage when light falls upon it. The two emitting light sources are at 660 nm red (visible), and at 800 nm infrared (not visible).

The tissues absorb light but enough is transmitted to reach the photodiode. The arrival of the arteriolar pulsation with oxygenated blood alters the amount of red and infrared light transmitted through to the finger. This change is calculated by a microprocessor and the amount of oxygenated blood in the tissue deduced. The size and the shape of the arteriolar pulsation is shown as a plethysmographic trace. You must be able to see a pulsatile trace to rely on the oximeter reading.

The sigmoid shape of the oxygen dissociation curve means that saturations of above 90% show adequate tissue oxygenation.

Oximetry is unreliable in the following instances:
- excessive movement
- venous congestion
- excessive illumination
- nail polish/false nails
- intravenous drugs: methylene blue, indocyanine green
- carbon monoxide poisoning

A low oxygen saturation (SpO_2 < 90%) demands an immediate response. Oxygenation of the tissues depends on the inspired oxygen concentration, lung function, haemoglobin concentration and cardiac output. The main causes of a low oxygen saturation are shown in Box 10.4. If necessary, deliver 100% oxygen to the lungs while determining the cause of the hypoxaemia and starting appropriate treatment.

Box 10.4 Causes of low oxygen saturation

- Oxygen supply
  - oxygen flow turned on?
  - machine delivering oxygen? (oxygen analyser)
  - vaporiser fault?
- Oxygen delivery to patient
  - circuit assembled correctly?
  - airway patent, NO OBSTRUCTION?
  - tracheal tube sited correctly?
  - DISCONNECTION?
- Lung function
  - normal airway pressure?
    - tracheal tube in right main bronchus?
    - bronchospasm?
  - pulmonary oedema, pneumothorax?
- Haemoglobin
  - unrecognised haemorrhage?
  - hypovolaemia?
- Heart
  - adequate blood pressure?
  - arrhythmias?
- Tissues
  - septicaemia?

The most common cause of a low oxygen saturation is an obstructed airway, and this should be excluded before other diagnoses are considered.

Capnography is used to measure carbon dioxide. This utilises the principle of infrared absorption. When infrared light falls on a molecule, it enhances the molecule's vibrational energy and the infrared light is absorbed by the molecule. The amount of infrared light absorbed at a specific wavelength is proportional to the amount of carbon dioxide present in the gas mixture.

In the presence of a stable cardiac output, arterial carbon dioxide tension is related inversely to alveolar ventilation:

$$P_aCO_2 \propto 1/V_A$$

Common causes of high and low P_aCO_2 are shown in Box 10.5.

Box 10.5 Common causes of high and low P_aCO_2

- Low
  - hyperventilation
  - low cardiac output: embolism (gas or blood)
- High
  - hypoventilation
  - rebreathing carbon dioxide: circuit failures
  - hypermetabolic states: malignant hyperthermia

Full monitoring equipment should be available in the recovery room, as well as in theatre. It must also be available for the transportation and transfer of patients.

10.4 Conclusion

The most important monitor during any anaesthetic procedure is the presence of a trained, vigilant anaesthetist. **Under no circumstances must you ever leave the theatre while a patient is under your care.**

Careful, repetitive clinical observation of the patient is the next essential procedure, followed by the appropriate use of monitors to assess the respiratory and cardiovascular system.

These principles apply to all surgical procedures. There are 'small operations' but there is no such thing as a 'small anaesthetic'.

Part II **Crises and complications**

As soon as you are capable of assessing and controlling the airway, ventilating the lungs and establishing vascular access, it is likely that you will be given a bleep. As the 'on-call' anaesthetist, your problems have now started, as you will be expected to assess and start the management of a large number of anaesthetic problems around the hospital.

In this section of the book we describe a variety of crises and complications. Some are common, such as cardiac arrest and massive haemorrhage, whereas others, such as malignant hyperthermia, are rare. Unfortunately, patients cannot be relied on to respect your lack of experience, and they have the uncanny habit of keeping the most unusual complications for the most junior members of staff at the most unsocial hours.

Some of the crises that develop in patients are caused by you, the anaesthetist. If you cause the crisis you must have the knowledge and skills to manage it.

Chapter 11 **Cardiac arrest**

It is imperative that you have a detailed knowledge of the management of cardiac arrest. In the operating theatre, and often on the wards, you will be responsible for making the decisions.

The causes of cardiac arrest in the operating theatre are broadly classified as follows:

- medical diseases
- surgical causes, especially haemorrhage (occult or massive) and occasionally vagal responses to surgical traction
- anaesthetic causes, especially hypoxia and hypercapnia from problems such as failure to secure the airway and ventilate the lungs and unnoticed disconnection of the anaesthetic circuit; also from technical disasters such as a tension pneumothorax after attempts at central venous cannulation.

11.1 Tracheal intubation

The tracheal tube must be correctly positioned and secured. When there is no cardiac output, no carbon dioxide is produced; the capnograph (which is normally not available in the ward) is thus valueless in assessing correct positioning of the tracheal tube. Visualisation of the tube passing through the laryngeal opening is critically important, and auscultation is used to ensure it is placed in the trachea and not the bronchus. The anaesthetist is the best person to do this. Don't let others do it!

The capnograph may be a guide to the adequacy of the cardiac output when cardiopulmonary resuscitation is undertaken.

How to Survive in Anaesthesia: A Guide for Trainees, Fourth Edition.
Neville Robinson, George Hall and William Fawcett.
© 2012 John Wiley & Sons, Ltd. Published 2012 by John Wiley & Sons, Ltd.

11.2 Defibrillation

Whenever you start to work in a new environment you must know where the defibrillator is kept and how it works. It should be tested every day without fail. A defibrillator is a capacitor and thus stores electrical charge. Usually, it has four controls:

• on
• charge
• defibrillate
• synchronisation

11.3 Oxygenation

It is essential that the lungs are ventilated with 100% oxygen. An oxygen analyser should be attached to the anaesthetic machine to confirm the nature of the fresh gas flow. (Check that the vaporisers are turned off.) If doubt exists, oxygen from a cylinder can be used.

11.4 Obstetrics

Fortunately, pregnant patients very rarely suffer from a cardiac arrest. If they do, you will see a severe case of 'obstetrician's distress' – an awesome sight. If the woman is less than 25 weeks pregnant, she can be treated as a non-pregnant adult. If she is more than 25 weeks pregnant, there are two priorities. First, the baby should be delivered immediately. Second, resuscitation must *not* occur with the patient in the supine position. The uterus will compress the inferior vena cava and inadequate venous return to the heart will result, with subsequent failure of patient resuscitation. Cardiopulmonary resuscitation should be made with the woman in a left lateral tilt to diminish caval compression. This can be achieved by a physical wedge, or by table tilt. A human wedge can be made by a member of the team kneeling on the floor and subsequently sitting on his/her heels. The woman is then positioned so that her back is on the thighs of the human wedge. Pregnant patients can be more difficult to intubate than non-pregnant women.

11.5 Adult resuscitation

In the UK the Resuscitation Council has issued guidelines for basic and advanced life support (Figures 11.1 and 11.2).

Adult Basic Life Support

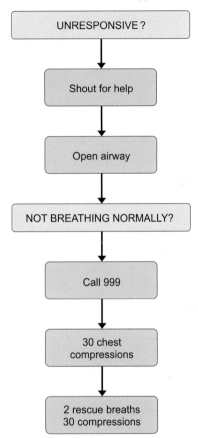

Figure 11.1 Adult basic life support algorithm. Reproduced with the kind permission of the Resuscitation Council (UK).

The potentially reversible causes of cardiac arrest are also listed in Figure 11.2 – these are known as the '4Hs and 4Ts'.

In adult basic life support it is important to ask for an automated external defibrillator (AED) if one is available. Remember to compress the chest to a depth of 5–6 cm at a rate of 100–120/minute. Do not stop CPR unless the patient shows signs of regaining vital signs. In advanced life support emphasis is again on the importance of minimal interruption in high-quality chest compressions. However, do not neglect the airway, and ensure that there is adequate oxygenation. When treating VF/VT cardiac arrest, adrenaline

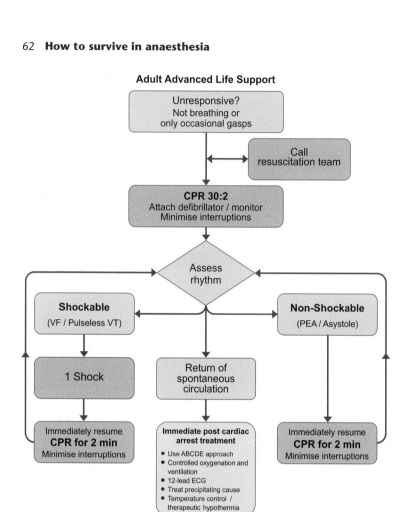

Adult Advanced Life Support

Unresponsive?
Not breathing or
only occasional gasps

Call
resuscitation team

CPR 30:2
Attach defibrillator / monitor
Minimise interruptions

Assess
rhythm

Shockable
(VF / Pulseless VT)

Non-Shockable
(PEA / Asystole)

1 Shock

Return of
spontaneous
circulation

Immediately resume
CPR for 2 min
Minimise interruptions

**Immediate post cardiac
arrest treatment**
• Use ABCDE approach
• Controlled oxygenation and
  ventilation
• 12-lead ECG
• Treat precipitating cause
• Temperature control /
  therapeutic hypothermia

Immediately resume
CPR for 2 min
Minimise interruptions

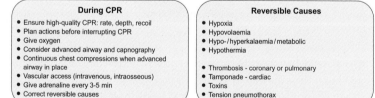

During CPR
• Ensure high-quality CPR: rate, depth, recoil
• Plan actions before interrupting CPR
• Give oxygen
• Consider advanced airway and capnography
• Continuous chest compressions when advanced
  airway in place
• Vascular access (intravenous, intraosseous)
• Give adrenaline every 3-5 min
• Correct reversible causes

Reversible Causes
• Hypoxia
• Hypovolaemia
• Hypo-/hyperkalaemia/metabolic
• Hypothermia

• Thrombosis - coronary or pulmonary
• Tamponade - cardiac
• Toxins
• Tension pneumothorax

Figure 11.2 Adult advanced life support algorithm. Reproduced with the kind permission of the Resuscitation Council (UK).

(epinephrine) 1 mg is given once chest compressions have restarted after the third shock and then every 3–5 minutes. Amiodarone 300 mg is also given after the third shock.

11.6 Arrhythmias

Two main types of arrhythmia occur in a cardiac arrest. These are non-shockable and shockable:
- non-shockable: pulseless electrical activity (PEA) – a QRS complex without a palpable pulse and asystole
- shockable: ventricular fibrillation (VF) or pulseless ventricular tachycardia (VT)

The core points of management are shown in Figure 11.2. The adult bradycardia and tachycardia algorithms are shown in Figures 11.3 and 11.4. These are becoming increasingly complex.

11.7 Paediatric resuscitation

The algorithms for basic and advanced paediatric life support are shown in Figures 11.5 and 11.6. The basic important features are:
- 5 initial rescue breaths
- a 15 : 2 chest compression : breath ratio
- a shock of 4 J/kg

11.8 Concentrations

Adrenaline (epinephrine) ampoules are available at concentrations of 1 in 1000 and 1 in 10,000. It is important that the amount of adrenaline present in 1 ml of each concentration is known, so that the correct doses can be given at a cardiac arrest.

$$1 : 1000 = 1 \text{ g in } 1000 \text{ ml}$$
$$= 1000 \text{ mg in } 1000 \text{ ml}$$
$$= 1 \text{ mg in } 1 \text{ ml}$$
$$1 : 10,000 = 1 \text{ g in } 10,000 \text{ ml}$$
$$= 1000 \text{ mg in } 10,000 \text{ ml} = 1 \text{ mg in } 10 \text{ ml}$$
$$= 1000 \text{ micrograms in } 10 \text{ ml}$$
$$= 100 \text{ micrograms in } 1 \text{ ml}$$

Therefore, there is 1 mg adrenaline in 1 ml of 1 in 1000, or in 10 ml of 1 in 10,000.

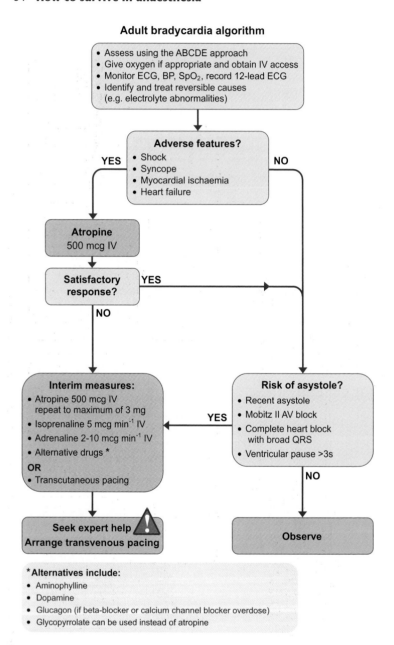

Figure 11.3 Adult bradycardia algorithm. Reproduced with the kind permission of the Resuscitation Council (UK).

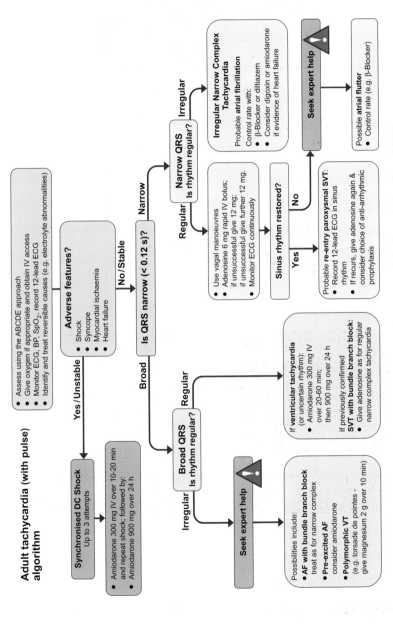

Figure 11.4 Adult tachycardia algorithm. Reproduced with the kind permission of the Resuscitation Council (UK).

Paediatric Basic Life Support
(Healthcare professionals with a duty to respond)

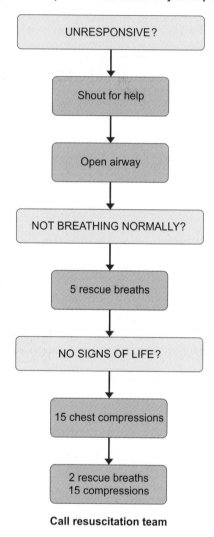

UNRESPONSIVE?

Shout for help

Open airway

NOT BREATHING NORMALLY?

5 rescue breaths

NO SIGNS OF LIFE?

15 chest compressions

2 rescue breaths
15 compressions

Call resuscitation team

Figure 11.5 Paediatric basic life support (healthcare professionals with a duty to respond). Reproduced with the kind permission of the Resuscitation Council (UK).

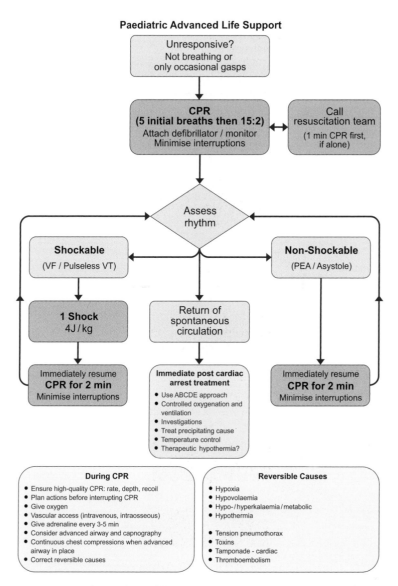

Figure 11.6 Paediatric advanced life support. Reproduced with the kind permission of the Resuscitation Council (UK).

11.9 Conclusion

The success rate of resuscitation in hospital, as assessed by the number of patients returning home, remains disappointing. The prompt recognition and management of the arrest is essential and, if it occurs during anaesthesia, the cause must be identified and treated.

The rapid establishment of ventilation of the lungs with oxygen and vascular access is essential for successful resuscitation.

Your anaesthetic skills often make you the natural leader of the arrest team.

Chapter 12 **Haemorrhage and blood transfusion**

12.1 Estimation of blood loss

Surgeons cause blood loss, and it is in their nature always to underestimate that loss. As an anaesthetist you must try to assess accurately the amount of blood shed and replace it with an appropriate intravenous solution. There are four main ways of estimating blood loss (Box 12.1).

Box 12.1 Blood loss estimation

- Clinical observation
- Weighing of swabs
- Volume of suction
- Dilution techniques

During surgery it is a useful exercise to try to guess how much blood has been lost before checking with the estimate derived from weighing the swabs and measuring the volume of suction. With practice, your guess will become reasonably accurate for a known surgeon. However, this method should not be relied on, and it can be hopelessly inaccurate when you start working with a new surgical team.

Apart from surgical spillage, it is important to remember that, in trauma, patients will have occult loss in limb and pelvic fractures, and in chest or abdominal injuries.

Swab weighing relies on the principle that 1 ml of blood weighs approximately 1 g. A 3 × 4 inch swab weighs 20 g when dry and about 35 g when saturated. This 15 g difference represents about 15 ml of blood. An 18 × 18 inch swab contains about 150 ml of blood when saturated. Three of these large

---

How to Survive in Anaesthesia: A Guide for Trainees, Fourth Edition.
Neville Robinson, George Hall and William Fawcett.
© 2012 John Wiley & Sons, Ltd. Published 2012 by John Wiley & Sons, Ltd.

swabs full of blood contain about 450 ml, which is equivalent to one unit of whole blood.

The volume of fluid in the suction apparatus may contain surgical 'washing fluid' as well as blood. This overestimate is a useful precaution, as the amount of blood on the surgical drapes, down the surgeons and on the floor cannot be measured. In major surgery it can easily be equivalent to 1–2 units of blood.

Dilution techniques are rarely used in clinical practice but rely on the measurement of the concentration of haemoglobin in the suction fluid to calculate the blood loss.

Patients should be transfused according to cardiovascular variables rather than relying on the estimates of blood loss. The heart rate, arterial pressure and central venous pressure are obvious guides, and the measurement of the haematocrit or haemoglobin may be useful. A haemoglobin concentration of 10 g/dl, or a haematocrit of 30%, is often considered the lower limit of adequate oxygen delivery, even when the circulating blood volume and cardiac output are maintained. Although this limit is arbitrary, we have found it a useful practical guide and will transfuse red cells unless there are obvious contraindications. Lower values of 25% haematocrit or 8 g/dl haemoglobin concentration have been proposed, but there is then little physiological reserve if further rapid blood loss occurs.

A cell saver system is used increasingly in major surgery to decrease the use of homologous blood.

12.2 Blood and blood products

Storage

Blood after donation is immediately cooled to 4–6 °C. These temperature limits must be rigidly observed to preserve the red cells and minimise the multiplication of chance bacterial contaminants. Blood from the refrigerator should be used within 30 minutes.

A unit (500 ml) of blood is collected into a bag that contains 70 ml of citrate, phosphate and dextrose (CPD) solution. The plasma is commonly centrifuged off for other use. The red cells are then suspended in a saline, adenine, glucose and mannitol (SAG-M) solution. The purpose of the storage additives is shown in Box 12.2.

Box 12.2 Additives used in red cell storage

- Citrate: chelates calcium
- Phosphate: maintains ATP, reduces haemolysis and increases red cell survival

- Saline: decreases viscosity of red cell concentrates
- Adenine: maintains ATP, improves red cell mobility
- Glucose: energy for red cells, decreases hydrolysis of ATP
- Mannitol: reduces haemolysis

Whole blood is devoid of functioning platelets after 2–3 days of storage and the clotting factors V and VIII are reduced to 10% of normal within 24 hours. Although adequate amounts of the coagulation factors I, II, VII, IX, X, XI, XII are present in whole blood, red cell concentrates contain virtually no coagulation factors.

Potassium concentrations rise progressively in stored blood and can reach up to 30 mmol/l after 3 weeks. Following transfusion, viable red cells re-establish their ionic pumping mechanism and intracellular uptake of potassium occurs rapidly. Blood $\geq$ 3 weeks old is acidic, with pH values down to 6.6, resulting mainly from the lactic acid generated by red cell metabolism.

Preparations

There are about 20 different types of blood and blood products available for adult and paediatric use. The main ones used by anaesthetists are shown in Table 12.1.

Table 12.1 Blood products in common use

Blood/blood product	Volume (ml) per unit	Storage temperature ($^\circ$C)	Shelf life
Whole blood	500	4–6	35 days
Red cell concentrates	300	4–6	35 days
Fresh frozen plasma	150	−30	1 year
Platelet concentrates	50	22	5 days
Cryoprecipitate	18	−30	1 year

Fresh frozen plasma (FFP) contains all the components of the coagulation, fibrinolytic and complement systems. In addition, it also has proteins that maintain oncotic pressure, fats and carbohydrates.

Cryoprecipitate contains factor VIII and fibrinogen.

Beriplex is a human prothrombin complex concentrate used for the emergency correction of oral anticoagulation with warfarin. It increases factors II, VII, IX, X and the anticoagulant inhibitors protein C and protein S.

12.3 Complications of blood transfusion

Complications of blood transfusion include those listed in Box 12.3.

Box 12.3 Blood transfusion complications

- Physical
  - circulatory overload
  - embolism (air, microaggregates)
  - hypothermia
- Immunological
  - pyrogenic
  - type I hypersensitivity
  - graft versus host reactions
- Biochemical
  - acid–base disturbances
  - hyperkalaemia
  - citrate toxicity
  - impaired oxygen release
- Infective
- Haemolytic transfusion reactions
- Disseminated intravascular coagulation

Physical

Circulatory overload should be avoided by the judicious transfusion of blood according to the measured cardiovascular variables such as arterial pressure, central venous pressure and heart rate. Air embolism can occur from errors in blood administration, particularly when the bags are pressurised. Microaggregates are platelet and white cell debris that are removed by the use of 20–40 μm blood filters. These filters are either screen or depth in nature. Reduced transfusion of microaggregates may result in a decreased incidence of non-haemolytic febrile reactions, and less pulmonary injury and histamine release. Depth filters cause impaction and absorption of microaggregates and screen filters operate by direct interception of the microemboli. Blood filters cause increased resistance to blood flow, haemolysis, complement activation, and can deplete the blood of any remaining viable platelets. We do not believe that their value has been proven and never use them.

Anaesthetised patients have impaired temperature regulation, and the rapid transfusion of cold blood exacerbates the hypothermia. The value of warming blood during transfusion has been demonstrated repeatedly, and this should be undertaken on every occasion.

Immunological

Pyrogenic reactions can occur in the recipient to white cell antigens or the polysaccharide products of bacterial metabolism. Rarely, stored blood contains Gram-negative bacteria. Plasma proteins are responsible for any anaphylactic or allergic reactions that happen. These reactions are rare, and range from severe hypotension to mild rashes. 'Graft versus host' reactions are caused by blood containing HLA-incompatible, immunocompetent lymphocytes being given to patients with immunosuppression. Pyrexia may develop, and the disease can be fatal without suitable transfusion precautions. The use of leucocyte-depleted red cell concentrates is expected to decrease the incidence of immunological complications.

It has been suggested, but is unproven, that patients with malignancy requiring transfusion have a greater risk of a recurrence.

Biochemical

The rapid infusion of large volumes of stored blood may result in acidosis in the recipient. This is particularly likely to occur if the liver is unable to metabolise the lactate and citrate because of inadequate hepatic perfusion, hypothermia or even hepatic disease. A persistent acidosis decreases myocardial function. A temporary improvement in cardiac output often follows the use of intravenous calcium chloride in these circumstances, although there is no obvious relationship to plasma ionised calcium values. The restoration of normal liver function usually corrects the problem.

Depletion of 2,3-diphosphoglycerate (DPG) in the red cells shifts the oxygen dissociation curve to the left and oxygen is released less easily from transfused blood. Modern additives have improved the concentration of 2,3-DPG for up to 14 days, and 25% of cells are back to normal function in 3 hours and 50% in 24 hours after transfusion.

Infective

All blood products except albumin and gamma globulin can transmit infectious diseases. Hepatitis B, C, syphilis and HIV are screened for, but cytomegalovirus, malaria, Epstein–Barr virus and parvovirus infection can be transmitted following transfusion.

Haemolytic transfusion reactions

Haemolytic and pyrogenic reactions are usually due to *errors* in the clerical administration of blood. However, blood group and rhesus incompatibility can also result in severe haemolytic reactions. Blood should be checked by two people against the patient's identity band. The recipient's name, hospital number, blood group and blood expiry date must be checked and signed for. In practice, during emergency work, it is often not possible for two people to check the blood and it is then *imperative that you slowly and deliberately check each unit.* Sometimes you have the opportunity to check all the blood before inducing anaesthesia.

Disseminated intravascular coagulation (DIC)

DIC is widespread activation of the coagulation and fibrinolytic systems, which results in clotting throughout the whole vasculature. It has many possible causes, but can occur in 30% of cases of massive transfusion. It presents primarily as a haemorrhagic disorder caused by loss of platelets and soluble clotting factors (especially fibrinogen).

12.4 Massive blood transfusion

Various definitions exist for this term. It is normally defined in one of three ways, based on volume and speed of replacement:
• acute administration of more than 1.5 times the estimated blood volume
• replacement of the patient's total blood volume by stored bank blood in less than 24 hours
• acute administration of more than 50% of the blood volume per hour
Formulae for estimating the blood volume are shown in Box 12.4.

Box 12.4 Blood volume formulae

• Neonate	90 ml/kg
• Infants 2 years of age	80 ml/kg
• Adult male	70 ml/kg
• Adult female	60 ml/kg

There is an increasing trend towards replacing all blood components at an early stage. This means that for every 2 units of blood consideration should be given to replacement with a pack of FFP and a pool of platelets. The aim is to prevent a coagulopathy rather than having to treat it.

It is recommended that, after a 4-unit transfusion, a set of basic screening tests is undertaken to exclude DIC. These are:
• haemoglobin and platelet count
• prothrombin time (PT) and activated partial thromboplastin time (APTT)
• plasma fibrinogen concentration
• fibrin degradation products
• pH from arterial blood gas analysis
The diagnosis of DIC is made by noting the trend:
• *increase*: APTT, PT, fibrin degradation products
• *decrease*: platelet count, fibrinogen concentration

The correction of these abnormalities is made after haematological consultation.

The abnormalities in PT and APTT are normally corrected by the administration of FFP (4 units). A low platelet count should be restored to above $100 \times 10^9/l$ by the administration of 6–8 units of platelets. Low fibrinogen levels are treated with cryoprecipitate, aiming for a level of less than 1 g/l (normal 2–4.5 g/l). If the patient has an arterial pH less than 7.2 and is continuing to bleed, the administration of 50 mmol bicarbonate (50 ml of 8.4% solution) should be considered. Recombinant activated factor VIIa can also be administered, if bleeding continues in spite of the use of FFP, platelets and cryoprecipitate.

In addition to laboratory tests to measure clotting, as shown above, 'near-patient' tests are also available. A thromboelastograph (TEG) provides quick (20–30 minute response) guidance on the state of the complete clotting cascade.

12.5 Checking blood for transfusion

Ensure that the blood to be transfused is compatible with the patient. There are several checks to stop incompatible blood being given to patients (Box 12.5). Do them carefully.

Box 12.5 Blood transfusion checks

- Blood product
  - check against label and compatibility and traceability tag
- Patient details
  - ensure identification details are the same on identity band, notes, compatibility and traceability tag
  - hospital number, first name, last name, date of birth, gender
    IN GENERAL ANAESTHESIA CONFIRM ALL THESE CAREFULLY: THE PATIENT IS UNCONSCIOUS AND FATAL MISMATCH ERRORS CAN OCCUR
- Blood group
  - ensure ABO and Rh D group and donation number are same on blood label and compatability and traceability tag
- Special requirements
  - gamma radiation or CMV-seronegative
- Expiry date the same on all labels and tags
- Inspect blood before use
  - leaks, evidence of haemolysis, discolouration or clots

12.6 Conclusion

Surgery results in blood loss. You must know how to estimate this loss, understand the blood products available and be able to use cardiovascular and haematological monitoring to transfuse them appropriately.

Think of blood as another potent drug that you will give frequently. It must be checked carefully before use, it can be life-saving, but it also has unwanted side effects.

The greatest disaster is to give the wrong blood to the patient. It is imperative that the blood is checked against the patient's identity band. **Never** check the blood bags solely with the transfusion form.

Chapter 13 **Anaphylactic reactions**

Although minor allergic reactions are not uncommon in anaesthesia, major anaphylactic reactions are rare. Prompt treatment, with the emphasis on the early use of adrenaline (epinephrine) will usually lead to a successful outcome.

Anaphylaxis is a severe, life-threatening, generalised or systemic hypersensitivity reaction. Histamine, serotonin and other vasoactive substances are liberated in response to an IgE-mediated reaction.

An anaphylactoid reaction results in the same clinical manifestations as an anaphylactic reaction, but is not mediated by a sensitising IgE antibody. Previous exposure to a drug will not have occurred, but susceptible individuals often have a history of allergies.

Every anaesthetist should know and practise an 'anaphylaxis drill'. The clinical manifestations of severe allergic reactions are shown in Box 13.1.

Box 13.1 Signs of severe allergic drug reactions

- Pruritis
- Flushing
- Erythema
- Coughing on induction of anaesthesia
- Nausea, vomiting and diarrhoea
- Angioedema
- Laryngeal oedema with stridor
- Bronchospasm with wheeze
- Hypotension
- Cardiovascular collapse – tachycardia or bradycardia
- Disseminated intravascular coagulation
- Sudden death

How to Survive in Anaesthesia: A Guide for Trainees, Fourth Edition.
Neville Robinson, George Hall and William Fawcett.
© 2012 John Wiley & Sons, Ltd. Published 2012 by John Wiley & Sons, Ltd.

The incidence of anaphylaxis is between 1 in 10,000 and 1 in 20,000 anaesthetics. It occurs more commonly in women than in men.

The majority of cases of anaphylaxis occurring during anaesthesia are caused by the neuromuscular blocking drugs. Latex allery is becoming increasingly common, with an onset typically 30–60 minutes after the start of surgery. Antibiotics continue to cause anaphylactic reactions, and it has been argued that they should always be given before induction of anaesthesia.

13.1 Treatment

The management of an anaphylactic reaction should be considered in two stages:
- immediate treatment
- secondary treatment

Immediate management (Box 13.2)

A reduction in peripheral vascular resistance and a loss of intravascular volume are the initial pathophysiological changes. Fluid therapy is important for resuscitation, and central venous pressure measurement may be necessary. However, the priority is intravenous adrenaline.

Box 13.2 Anaphylaxis – immediate management

- Use ABC approach and work as a team
- Stop administration of suspected drug, if possible
- Call for HELP and note time
- Stop anaesthesia and surgery, if feasible. Unconsciousness can be maintained with inhalational agent
- Maintain airway
- Give *100% oxygen* (consider intubation and ventilation)
- Give intravenous *adrenaline* (especially if bronchospasm present):
    - 0.5–1.0 ml of 1:10,000 (50–100 µg)
    - 5–8 µg/min if prolonged therapy required
    - children 1.0 µg/kg
- Repeat bolus of adrenaline as necessary
- Start intravascular volume replacement by colloid or crystalloid 10 ml/kg
- Consider CPR
- Transfer patient to appropriate critical care area

Secondary management (Box 13.3)

Intensive care facilities may be needed. Awareness can occur and should be prevented.

Box 13.3 Anaphylaxis – secondary management

- Adrenaline-resistant bronchospasm. Consider:
  - intravenous salbutamol 250 μg loading dose and 5–20 μg/min maintenance, *or*
  - aminophylline 4–8 mg/kg over 20 minutes
- Bronchospasm and/or cardiovascular collapse. Consider:
  - intravenous hydrocortisone 200 mg, *or*
  - methyl prednisolone 2 g
- Antihistamines. Consider:
  - intravenous chlorpheniramine 10 mg diluted, administer slowly
- After 20 minutes and severe acidosis present. Consider:
  - sodium bicarbonate (25–50 ml 8.4%)
- Catecholamine infusions. Consider:
  - adrenaline 5 mg in 500 ml (10 μg/ml) at rate 10–85 ml/h, *or*
  - noradrenaline 4 mg in 500 ml (8 μg/ml) at rate 25–100 ml/h
- Consider coagulopathy: clotting screen
- Arterial gas analysis for oxygenation and degree of acidosis
- Do not extubate until airway safe

13.2 Investigations

After a severe allergic drug reaction, the patient must be investigated thoroughly and both the patient and the general practitioner informed of the results. This is usually carried out in consultation with a clinical immunologist. The investigations normally take place in the following order:

1 blood tests for confirmation of allergic reaction
2 full anaesthetic history
3 skin tests
4 patient reporting: hazard card, MedicAlert bracelet

At the time of the reaction, and 1, 2 and 24 hours later, serial blood samples (5–10 ml clotted blood) are taken for tryptase (a neutral protease released from mast cells), complement activation, and IgE antibody concentrations. These will confirm that a reaction has occurred, but will not identify the causative agent.

Ensure that you liaise with the hospital laboratory staff: the samples are precious.

After a full medical history and a delay of at least 4 weeks, a 'skin prick test' is undertaken. This correctly identifies most causative agents. Full resuscitation equipment must be available, and detailed protocols have been described, indicating appropriate dilutions of drugs and the use of control solutions.

The case must be reported to the MHRA (Medicines and Healthcare Products Regulatory Agency) in the UK. The patient should carry a written record of the reaction and either an anaesthetic hazard card or a MedicAlert bracelet.

13.3 Conclusion

Life-threatening anaphylaxis is a rare complication of anaesthesia.

A knowledge of the immediate and secondary management must be learnt during the early months of training.

The mainstay of immediate treatment is intravenous adrenaline. Remember:

ANAPHYLAXIS = ADRENALINE (EPINEPHRINE)

Chapter 14 **Malignant hyperthermia**

Malignant hyperthermia (MH) is a rare complication of general anaesthesia that results from an abnormal increase in muscle metabolism in response to all potent inhalational agents and suxamethonium. There is often a family history of death or major problems associated with anaesthesia, and the gene is inherited as an autosomal dominant. Even with the ready availability of a specific therapeutic drug, dantrolene, deaths from MH still occur, mostly because of a failure to recognise the onset of the syndrome. If you are lucky, you will never see a patient with MH, but we know an anaesthetist who induced MH in three patients within five years! The main reason why this rare syndrome provokes so much attention is because, like anaphylaxis, it is one of those occasions when an anaesthetic drug can kill the patient.

The primary defect in MH is in calcium homeostasis within the sarcoplasmic reticulum of skeletal muscle. Abnormal increases in calcium ion concentration occur on exposure to triggering agents, and this biochemical change results in acidosis, heat production and muscle stiffness.

Estimates of the incidence of MH vary, but a figure of 1 in 100,000 is commonly cited. This value represents typical practice in a district general hospital, but there is an increased incidence in the following groups:
- males
- children and young adults
- patients with congenital musculoskeletal disorders

Thus, if you work in a major orthopaedic centre, which undertakes scoliosis surgery in adolescents, you are more likely to encounter the problem.

It is helpful to try to identify MH before surgery by noting the following points:
- family history of problems or sudden death associated with general anaesthesia

---

How to Survive in Anaesthesia: A Guide for Trainees, Fourth Edition.
Neville Robinson, George Hall and William Fawcett.
© 2012 John Wiley & Sons, Ltd. Published 2012 by John Wiley & Sons, Ltd.

- increased circulating creatine kinase (CK) concentration
- *in vitro* testing of muscle biopsy to caffeine and halothane

Unfortunately, circulating CK concentrations are of limited use. They may be normal in MH-susceptible patients, and there are many other causes of an increased CK concentration. Nevertheless, if there is a family history of MH and the patient has an abnormally raised CK without obvious cause, they are likely to be MH-susceptible. *In vitro* testing of a muscle biopsy is, at present, the most accurate method of diagnosing MH, but it is undertaken only in specialised centres. The patient is described as MHS (susceptible), MHN (normal), or MHE (equivocal). MHE means that they respond positively to either halothane or caffeine, but not both.

MH is triggered by all volatile anaesthetic drugs and suxamethonium. The response to the administration of suxamethonium at induction of anaesthesia is abnormal in some MH-susceptible patients. Instead of the usual fasciculations followed by muscle relaxation, there are vigorous fasciculations with failure to relax and, in particular, masseter spasm. This spasm makes opening the mouth difficult, and so tracheal intubation may be a problem. The occurrence of masseter spasm should be treated as an important prognostic indicator of possible MH susceptibility (approximately 50%).

Management is undertaken as shown below:

1 HELP
2 Halt anaesthesia
3 Do not give volatile agents
4 Elective surgery: abandon and monitor patient
5 Emergency surgery:
   - follow advice
   - monitor patient
   - use 'safe' techniques (see Section 14.3 below)
   - prepare to treat MH
   - perform arterial gas analysis early and regularly

The key feature is *not to administer potent volatile agents*. Suxamethonium alone usually results in a relatively mild, self-limiting MH, whereas the combination of suxamethonium with a volatile anaesthetic is a potent trigger.

14.1 Presentation

There are no obvious signs of the onset of MH, other than an abnormal response to suxamethonium. The main clinical signs are shown in Box 14.1.

Box 14.1   Clinical signs of malignant hyperthermia (MH)

- Abnormal response to suxamethonium (masseter spasm)
- Tachycardia (possibly arrhythmias)
- Tachypnoea
- Increased use of sodalime
- Peripheral cyanosis
- Muscle stiffness
- Patient feels hot

The peripheral circulation is often decreased in MH, due to the marked increase in catecholamine secretion, so do not wait for the brow to feel hot – it may never happen! The metabolic signs of MH are more obvious, and reflect the massive stimulation of muscle metabolism (Box 14.2).

Box 14.2   Metabolic signs of malignant hyperthermia

- Acidosis
  - increased CO_2 production
  - increased lactic acid production
- Hyperkalaemia
- Haemoconcentration
- Hyperglycaemia
- Hypoxaemia
- Hyperthermia

The earliest objective sign of the onset of MH is increased CO_2 production as shown by a raised end-tidal CO_2 concentration with capnography. Body temperature is not a reliable sign, unless a good estimate of core temperature is available (not rectal). The metabolic changes provide the basis for the confirmation of the suspected diagnosis. Arterial gas analysis should be undertaken, and in established MH it will show a severe acidosis, both respiratory and metabolic, and often hyperkalaemia.

Once the diagnosis of MH has been confirmed, then correct treatment must be started immediately.

14.2 Treatment

The treatment of MH can be considered as specific therapy with dantrolene and general supportive management (Box 14.3).

Box 14.3 Overall management plan for malignant hyperthermia

- Specific treatment
  - dantrolene
- General supportive therapy
  - acidosis
  - hyperkalaemia
  - haemoconcentration
  - arrhythmias
  - hyperthermia

Dantrolene must be administered promptly. The following guidelines have been found to be effective:

1 Discontinue volatile agents and terminate surgery, if possible.
2 Hyperventilate with 100% O_2 (2–3 times minute volume). Use opioid + benzodiazepine to maintain unconsciousness, or propofol infusion.
3 Correct metabolic acidosis (at least 100 mmol bicarbonate).
4 Dantrolene 1 mg/kg intravenously every 10 min until MH controlled. Assess therapy by:
   - arterial gas analysis
   - tachycardia
   - muscle stiffness
   - temperature
5 Establish appropriate monitoring.
6 Correct hyperkalaemia and rehydrate.
7 Treat severe tachycardia (small dose of beta-blocker).
8 Cool if necessary (infants and children only).
9 Induce diuresis when rehydrated.
10 Monitor carefully for 24 hours (ICU).

Dantrolene is difficult to dissolve and it can take a long time to form a solution. Once it is in suspension, use it. Fortunately, dantrolene works rapidly, and 1 mg/kg is often sufficient to stop the hypermetabolism within a few minutes. Most patients require a total dose of only 1–2 mg/kg.

Do not waste time on cooling the patient unless it is an infant or child; thermogenesis will cease once the MH is controlled.

14.3 Anaesthesia for MH-susceptible patients

It is much easier to manage MH if you are aware of the problem before the anaesthetic. A 'safe' technique means avoiding the potent volatile agents and suxamethonium and using a 'clean' anaesthetic machine. This is obtained by removing the vaporisers, changing all disposable tubing and then purging the machine with 10 litres of O_2 for 10 minutes. Regional or general anaesthesia may be used (Box 14.4).

Box 14.4 Anaesthesia in suspected malignant hyperthermia

- Regional anaesthesia
  - all drugs safe
- General anaesthesia
  - premedication: benzodiazepine, opioids
  - induction: all intravenous drugs safe
  - neuromuscular blockade: all non-depolarising drugs safe
  - maintenance: N_2O-O_2 – total intravenous anaesthesia

Full monitoring must be undertaken – capnography, oxygen consumption, temperature measurement and often the intravascular measurement of arterial pressure and central venous pressure.

14.4 Conclusion

Malignant hyperthermia is not easy to diagnose. Although it is rare, the possibility of MH must be considered if you find an unexpected increase in CO_2 excretion, tachycardia or tachypnoea during anaesthesia. The diagnosis is confirmed by arterial gas analysis.

Dantrolene is effective if given early. Know where it is kept in theatre – one day you may need it urgently.

Chapter 15 **Local anaesthetic toxicity**

Local anaesthetic agents are used to provide intra- and postoperative analgesia. Intraoperatively they can be used as the sole analgesic for surgery, but they are commonly used with sedation or in combination with general anaesthesia.

Lignocaine (lidocaine) and bupivacaine are the most popular local anaesthetic drugs. Ropivacaine and L-bupivacaine are also available and have variable popularity. The choice of drug depends on the speed of onset, the total amount of drug needed and the duration of action required. The characteristics of the commonly used drugs are shown in Table 15.1.

Table 15.1 Characteristics of local anaesthetic drugs

Agent	Duration (h)	Plain (mg/kg)	With adrenaline (mg/kg)
		Maximum dose	
Lignocaine	1–3	3	7
Bupivacaine	1–4	2	2
L-Bupivacaine	2–6	2	2
Ropivacaine	1–6	3	3

Adrenaline (epinephrine) is sometimes added to the local anaesthetic agent to prolong its use, and to decrease the vascularity of the operative field (for example, in thyroid surgery). It must not be used in proximity to terminal arterioles or arteries, as an adequate collateral arterial supply is not available to perfuse distal tissues, and ischaemia will occur. The recommendations for the safe use of adrenaline are listed in Box 15.1.

How to Survive in Anaesthesia: A Guide for Trainees, Fourth Edition.
Neville Robinson, George Hall and William Fawcett.
© 2012 John Wiley & Sons, Ltd. Published 2012 by John Wiley & Sons, Ltd.

Box 15.1 Recommendations for the safe use of adrenaline in local anaesthetic solutions

• No hypoxia
• No hypercarbia
• Caution with arrhythmogenic volatile agents
• Concentration of $\leq$ 1 : 200,000
• Dose less than 20 ml of 1 : 200,000 in 10 min
• Total dose less than 30 ml/h

Occasionally, the anaesthetist is responsible for supervising the preparation of a 1 : 200,000 adrenaline solution. The commonly available dilutions of adrenaline are 1 : 1000 and 1 : 10,000. Therefore, either:

1 ml of 1 : 10,000 adrenaline diluted to a total volume of
20 ml = 1 : 200,000 solution

or

0.1 ml of 1 : 1000 adrenaline diluted to a total volume of
20 ml = 1 : 200,000 solution

The former is more accurate, as measuring 0.1 ml is not easy. A similar calculation to that described in Chapter 11 shows that 1 ml of 1 : 200,000 adrenaline solution contains 5 µg adrenaline.

15.1 What does the term 'percentage' mean?

Local anaesthetic drugs come in vials displaying the percentage concentration contained. The word 'percentage' means grams in 100 ml. The maximum dose of local anaesthetic can be calculated as follows. For example, if you are using 1% plain lignocaine in an 80 kg patient:

1% = 1 gram in 100 ml, which is
1000 mg in 100 ml, which is
10 mg in 1 ml

The maximum dose of lignocaine is 3 mg/kg (Table 15.1) so the patient can have a total of 3 × 80 mg = 240 mg. As there are 10 mg/ml the total dose is 24 ml 1% plain lignocaine. Similar calculations can be made for other concentrations.

The maximum dose should not be exceeded when these drugs are used subcutaneously, as toxicity may occur. The administration of local anaesthetics accidentally into veins or arteries will also cause anaesthetic toxicity.

Toxicity is rare, but two of the authors have induced convulsions in patients while injecting local anaesthetics. Toxicity can be mild or severe.

15.2 Signs and symptoms of mild toxicity

The signs of mild toxicity are shown in Box 15.2. A patient with mild toxicity must be observed carefully in case severe toxicity occurs. Stop administering the drug and monitor the patient with an ECG. Mild symptoms usually resolve quickly when drug administration ceases, but severe toxicity can develop.

Box 15.2 Signs of mild local anaesthetic toxicity

- Anxiety
- Restlessness
- Nausea
- Tinnitus
- Perioral tingling
- Tremor
- Tachypnoea

15.3 Signs and symptoms of severe toxicity

The signs of severe toxicity (Box 15.3) may occur at the time of injection of the local anaesthetic but also up to 20 minutes after the drug has been injected. Surgeons may inadvertently cause toxicity when performing operations under local anaesthesia or when injecting local anaesthetics at the end of surgery. Anaesthetists can cause toxicity from topping up epidural analgesia inappropriately and when performing specific nerve blocks. It is important to remember that the cardiac toxic effects of local anaesthetics, especially bupivacaine, are very hard to reverse and prolonged treatment of a patient with local anaesthetic toxicity is needed.

Box 15.3 Signs of severe local anaesthetic toxicity

- Sudden alteration in mental state with agitation or loss of consciousness, with or without tonic–clonic convulsions
- Cardiovascular collapse
  - sinus bradycardia
  - conduction blocks
  - ventricular arrhythmias
  - asystole

15.4 Treatment of severe local anaesthetic toxicity

Intralipid should be stored in the theatres and you should know where it is. The immediate management of toxicity is shown in Boxes 15.4, 15.5 and 15.6.

Box 15.4 Immediate management of severe local anaesthetic toxicity

- Stop injecting the local anaesthetic
- Call for help
- Maintain airway with 100% oxygen
- Anaesthetist may need to intubate trachea to secure the airway
- Intravenous access
- Control seizures by diazepam bolus 5 mg, thiopentone, propofol or magnesium 4 g slowly
- Assess cardiovascular status throughout

Box 15.5 Treatment of severe local anaesthetic toxicity without circulatory arrest

- Treat hypotension, bradycardia and arrhythmias conventionally
- Consider intravenous lipid emulsion
  - start intravenous infusion of 20% lipid emulsion at 15 ml/kg/h
  - increase to 30 ml/kg/h after 5 min if cardiovascular or clinical deterioration
  - do not exceed a total dose of 12 ml/kg
- Propofol is not a substitute
- Lignocaine should not be given to treat arrhythmias

Box 15.6 Management of cardiac arrest associated with local anaesthetic injection

- Start CPR as per guidelines
- Manage arrhythmias using the same guidelines; they may be refractory to treatment
- Prolonged resuscitation may be necessary
- Treat with lipid emulsion
  - bolus intravenous Intralipid 20% 1.5 ml/kg over 1 min
  - repeat this bolus injection twice at 5-minute intervals
  - a maximum of 3 doses can be given
- Recovery from cardiac arrest may take 1 hour
- If facilities are available, cardiopulmonary bypass may be needed

Success is dependent on a prompt diagnosis and prolonged treatment of the patient. Follow-up includes transfer to a critical care area until recovery has occurred. Tests to exclude iatrogenic pancreatitis should be undertaken for 2 days.

15.5 Conclusion

Local anaesthetic toxicity is rare but can kill! Know the safe doses of drugs, aspirate prior to injection to avoid intravascular administration, and give all local anaesthetics slowly. Resuscitation, if severe toxicity occurs, can take several hours.

Chapter 16 **Stridor – upper airway obstruction**

Acute stridor is a life-threatening emergency. It usually occurs in children, but is occasionally found in adults. Complete obstruction of the upper airway may occur rapidly, and the change from partial to complete obstruction is often unpredictable. Upper airway obstruction will lead to fatigue and respiratory failure if left untreated, and pulmonary oedema may result from prolonged airway obstruction.

The common causes of airway obstruction are shown in Box 16.1. Laryngospasm and post-intubation oedema are considered in Chapter 18.

Box 16.1 Common causes of upper airway obstruction

- Congenital
- Acquired
  - infective
    - laryngotracheobronchitis (croup)
    - epiglottitis
  - traumatic
    - burns/smoke inhalation
    - foreign body inhalation
    - post-intubation laryngospasm/oedema
  - neoplastic

16.1 Clinical presentation

Inspiratory stridor occurs when the obstruction is at or above the level of the cricoid ring. Expiratory stridor, wheeze and chest hyperinflation are found with lower intrathoracic obstruction (for example, foreign body).

How to Survive in Anaesthesia: A Guide for Trainees, Fourth Edition.
Neville Robinson, George Hall and William Fawcett.
© 2012 John Wiley & Sons, Ltd. Published 2012 by John Wiley & Sons, Ltd.

Stridor is seen initially on exertion but, as the obstruction worsens, it occurs at rest. Children often prefer to sit, and there is hyperextension of the neck in an effort to prevent airway collapse. Chest recession and the use of the accessory muscles of respiration occur. Drooling results from a failure to swallow saliva. There is a gradual loss of interest in the surroundings and also a reduced level of consciousness (Box 16.2).

Box 16.2 Symptoms and signs of upper airway obstruction

- Type of stridor: inspiratory/expiratory
- Barking cough
- Hoarseness
- Chest recession
- Accessory muscle usage
- Sitting-forwards position
- Nasal flaring
- Hyperextension of neck
- Drooling
- Tachycardia
- Tachypnoea
- Cyanosis
- Loss of interest
- Reduced consciousness

16.2 Diagnosis

A concise and relevant history with repeated, frequent examinations of the child should be made. A past history of *Haemophilus influenzae* type b (Hib) vaccination makes epiglottitis an unlikely, but not impossible, diagnosis. Quiet observation of the child from a distance will often provide all the necessary information. A chest x-ray film is rarely necessary and *should only be done in the intensive care unit*, as appropriate resuscitation facilities must be available. This usually precludes the radiology department at night.

Examination of the child is difficult and may be unreliable. Exhaustion happens rapidly. Cyanosis is often difficult to detect and is an indication for urgent transfer to an intensive care unit. Children should also be assessed regarding the amount of stridor, sternal retraction, tachypnoea and tachycardia they have.

Pulse oximetry (more than 94% saturation on air) may confirm adequate oxygenation but arterial gas analysis is unhelpful. It will certainly upset the child, exacerbate the condition, and may delay treatment. If you have any doubts about the severity of the obstruction, admit the child to the intensive care unit and accompany the child yourself.

Laryngotracheobronchitis (croup)

Croup affects the whole respiratory tract, but oedema of the glottic and subglottic region causes the airway obstruction. The aetiology is:
* viral parainfluenza, respiratory syncytial, mycoplasmic pneumonia
* bacterial
* spasmodic

The child (mean age about 18 months) usually has a history of an upper respiratory tract infection with moderate fever for 48 hours before the onset of stridor.

Stridor is often worse at night, and stridor at rest is an indication for hospital admission.

The principles of care are:
1 Give adequate hydration.
2 Give paracetamol elixir 15 mg/kg every 6 hours.
3 Give nebulised adrenaline (epinephrine) 0.5 ml/kg 1 : 1000 (maximum 5 ml) every 1–4 hours depending on severity. Monitor with ECG.
4 Worsening respiratory distress, reduced consciousness and failure to respond to adrenaline is an indication for tracheal intubation.
5 Steroids decrease the duration of intubation.

Bacterial tracheitis, commonly from *Staphylococcus aureus*, requires antibiotic treatment (for example, cefotaxime 50 mg/kg every 6 hours). Spasmodic croup occurs suddenly at night without a pre-existing infection. There is a dramatic response to nebulised adrenaline, and dexamethasone 0.6 mg/kg is also effective.

Epiglottitis

This is caused mainly by *Haemophilus influenzae* type b infection and occurs in the 2–7-year-old group.

The incidence has declined dramatically since vaccination programmes have been implemented. The history is typically short. There is a high fever, malaise, dysphagia, dysphonia, an absent cough, and the stridor has a unique, low-pitched, snoring quality. The child will sit with an open mouth. Antibiotic therapy should be started and, if there is a high risk of obstruction, an artificial airway should be inserted. If complete obstruction occurs before intubation, hand ventilation is usually possible despite the oedematous structures.

Foreign body

Some foreign bodies will pass down into the bronchi, usually the right, but others will lodge in the larynx, causing obstruction and the risk of hypoxic arrest. The European Resuscitation Council recommends the following treatment:

- *Infants less than 1 year*: five back blows between shoulder blades with the head lower than the trunk and the child prone. If this does not work, five chest thrusts with the child supine can be given.
- *Children more than 1 year*: if the above is unsuccessful, then abdominal thrusts with the child supine (Heimlich manoeuvre) can be performed.

In a life-threatening situation, a foreign body in the laryngeal area can be removed under direct vision using a laryngoscope and a pair of Magill intubating forceps. This should be attempted only by an experienced anaesthetist.

16.3 Management of intubation

If a child is deteriorating, or unresponsive to treatment, tracheal intubation to bypass the obstruction must be undertaken.

The principles of management are as follows:

1 Get HELP: an *experienced anaesthetist* is needed.
2 ENT surgeon should be present if possible. ? Tracheostomy.
3 Transfer the child to theatre/intensive care unit.
4 Supervise transfer and take resuscitation equipment.
5 Keep parents present and informed.
6 Induce anaesthesia via inhalational route: oxygen and sevoflurane.
7 Insert intravenous cannula *after* induction.
8 Give atropine 20 µg/kg intravenously.
9 Monitor fully.
10 Use full range of tracheal tubes – smaller than expected for age.
11 Secure tracheal tube. ? Change to nasal.
12 Transfer from theatre to intensive care unit if necessary.
13 ? Sedate child.
14 Humidify inspired gases.
15 Maintain good airway toilet.

It is important not to upset the child, as this may precipitate complete obstruction of the airway, and for this reason intravenous cannulation should not be attempted until after induction of anaesthesia.

A principle of anaesthesia that is *absolute* is that neuromuscular blocking drugs must *not* be used if there are any doubts about the patency of the upper airway (ability to ventilate the lungs) or the ease of intubation. A patient who is impossible to ventilate and intubate will die of hypoxia if he/she is paralysed. In this situation tracheal intubation must be undertaken using either local anaesthetic techniques or inhalational anaesthesia. If an inhalational technique is used, it is imperative that intubation is not attempted until deep anaesthesia has been achieved. Alternatively the airway may be secured by a tracheostomy or cricothyroid puncture. In children with upper airway obstruction, inhalational anaesthesia is the chosen method, and this may take up to 15 minutes.

Atropine is given to block the bradycardia that may occur during intubation. The tracheal tube must not be allowed to come out, as this causes much excitement amongst the staff! It should be well secured to prevent an alert child from pulling it out unexpectedly – children are often sedated.

The tracheal tube can be removed when the child has recovered from the infection and there is a leak around the tube indicating that the oedema has subsided.

16.4 Conclusion

Stridor is a medical emergency that needs assistance from an experienced anaesthetist. A trainee must know the principles of maintaining a patent airway in this situation. If you have any doubts about the severity of the obstruction, transfer the child to an intensive care unit and accompany him or her on transfer. Stay calm – you are dealing with a frightened child, very worried parents and a paediatrician who often knows less about an obstructed airway than you.

Chapter 17 **Pneumothorax**

A pneumothorax is the presence of air within the pleural cavity. For it to occur, a communication must be present between the pleural cavity and either the tracheobronchial tree or the atmosphere by a defect in the chest wall. The main causes are shown in Box 17.1.

Box 17.1 Causes of pneumothorax

- Spontaneous
  - asthma
  - Marfan's syndrome
- Iatrogenic
  - central venous catheters
  - surgery (for example, nephrectomy)
- Traumatic
  - fractured ribs
  - other thoracic trauma

An emergency arises when a *tension pneumothorax* develops. This is most likely to occur when intermittent positive pressure ventilation is applied to the lungs of patients with the following problems:

- undiagnosed spontaneous pneumothorax
- emphysema
- lung bullae
- asthma

It is important to remember that *all* patients have the potential to develop a pneumothorax in anaesthesia. The situation is exacerbated by the fact that

---

How to Survive in Anaesthesia: A Guide for Trainees, Fourth Edition.
Neville Robinson, George Hall and William Fawcett.
© 2012 John Wiley & Sons, Ltd. Published 2012 by John Wiley & Sons, Ltd.

nitrous oxide diffuses rapidly into gas-filled spaces and thus increases the size of any pneumothorax.

In a tension pneumothorax, air entering the pleural cavity is unable to return to the lung and increases the pressure in the hemithorax, causing lung collapse. The mediastinum is shifted across the midline, decreasing venous return and impeding cardiac output, with impaired ventilation to the other lung. This combination of major physiological changes is potentially lethal.

The diagnosis is not easy, but should be suspected when the signs shown in Box 17.2 occur during or shortly after anaesthesia.

Box 17.2 Signs of pneumothorax in anaesthesia

- Unexplained cyanosis
- Wheeze
- 'Silent' chest on auscultation
- Difficulty with ventilation
- High airway pressures
- Sudden change in airway pressures
- Tachycardia
- Hypotension

17.1 Treatment

If time allows, a chest x-ray film in expiration will confirm the diagnosis. Ultrasound may also be used. Nitrous oxide should be discontinued. A chest drain must be inserted. In a life-threatening situation a 14 gauge cannula should be inserted into the pleural cavity to relieve the tension pneumothorax. This must then be connected to an underwater drainage system.

A chest drainage tube is inserted into the second intercostal space in the midclavicular line or the fifth intercostal space in the midaxillary line. It is important to insert the tube through a *high* intercostal space.

One author managed to place a right-sided chest drain using the transhepatic route, which was associated with a spectacular blood loss. Prompt surgery saved the patient. The important features of inserting a chest drain are stated below.

1 Use an aseptic technique.
2 If patient is unanaesthetised, inject local anaesthetic from skin to periosteum.
3 Make 2–3 cm horizontal incision.

4 Make blunt dissection through the tissues until it is just over the top of the rib.

5 Puncture the parietal pleural with the tip of a clamp and put a gloved finger into the incision to avoid injury to any organs and to clear the area of any adhesions or clots.

6 Clamp end of tube and advance it through the pleura to the desired length.

7 Connect tube to chest drain – the underwater tube should be placed below 5 cm into the water to minimise resistance.

8 Suture the tube in place and confirm position by a chest x-ray film.

17.2 Conclusion

Pneumothorax is uncommon in anaesthesia but must be considered when certain signs arise unexpectedly during or after anaesthesia. It is particularly likely in operations in the renal area. A tension pneumothorax must be treated by the insertion of a chest drain or, if this is unavailable, a 14 gauge intravenous cannula may be used temporarily.

Chapter 18 **Common intraoperative problems**

Problems occurring during anaesthesia and surgery must be considered in an appropriate way. For example, the onset of an arrhythmia during surgery may have an anaesthetic cause, or it may result from surgical stimulation.

A disturbance of cardiac rhythm is not necessarily indicative of myocardial disease. If the arrhythmia is accompanied by sweating and hypertension it probably results from excessive sympathoadrenal activity.

You must learn to consider the causation of intraoperative problems in the following order:

- anaesthetic
- surgical
- medical

In particular, we recommend that the following safety check is undertaken whenever an unexpected problem arises:

- Is the anaesthetic machine working correctly?
- Are the gas flows correct?
- Is the circuit assembled correctly and working?
- Is the airway patent?

This fundamental principle of an anaesthetic cause, before a surgical cause, before a medical cause, cannot be overemphasised. The simple mechanistic approach that a bradycardia needs intravenous atropine will be fatal if the slow heart rate is a response to hypoxaemia following a disconnection within the circuit. Identifying the site of the disconnection and oxygenating the patient is the obvious priority. Common causes of intraoperative problems are shown in Box 18.1.

How to Survive in Anaesthesia: A Guide for Trainees, Fourth Edition.
Neville Robinson, George Hall and William Fawcett.
© 2012 John Wiley & Sons, Ltd. Published 2012 by John Wiley & Sons, Ltd.

Box 18.1 Common causes of intraoperative problems

- Anaesthetic
  - exclude HYPOXIA
  - exclude HYPERCAPNIA
  - response to laryngoscopy and intubation?
  - correct gas flow settings?
  - correct use of volatile agents?
  - pain?
  - awareness?
  - drugs correct? interactions?
  - adequate monitoring?
  - malignant hyperthermia?
- Surgical
  - reflex responses – eye, dental surgery, vagal stimulation?
  - retractors correctly sited?
  - haemorrhage – occult?
- Medical
  - specific diseases – cardiac?
  - undiagnosed disease – phaeochromocytoma?
  - electrolyte imbalance?
  - acid–base balance?

Some problems remain after anaesthetic and surgical causes have been eliminated, and these need specific treatment.

18.1 Laryngospasm

Reflex closure of the glottis from spasm of the vocal cords is usually due to laryngeal stimulation. Common causes include insertion of a Guedel airway or laryngoscope, the presence of a tracheal tube and secretions in the airway. It can also arise as a response to surgical stimulation in a lightly anaesthetised patient. Thus, it occurs not only on induction of anaesthesia but also intraoperatively, and occasionally postoperatively.

The airway obstruction can lead to hypoxia and, in severe cases, pulmonary oedema can result.

Treatment
The management of laryngospasm depends on its severity, as shown in Box 18.2.

Box 18.2 Management of laryngospasm

1 Identify stimulus and remove, if possible
2 Give 100% O_2 and get help
3 Ensure patent airway
4 Tighten expiratory valve to apply a positive airway pressure to 'break' the spasm and increase O_2 intake with each breath (BE CAREFUL)
5 Consider deepening anaesthesia with an induction agent such as propofol
6 If unable to ventilate, give suxamethonium, tracheal intubation, and deepen anaesthesia. Ensure intubation and ventilation is feasible

---

There is a belief that a patient with severe laryngospasm and cyanosis will gasp a breath just before hypoxaemia is fatal. Do not try to verify this tenet – if in doubt paralyse and ventilate the patient.

18.2 Wheeze

Wheeziness during anaesthesia may be caused by many factors other than bronchospasm (Box 18.3). These causes must be eliminated before treatment for bronchospasm is started.

Box 18.3 Differential diagnoses of wheeze

- Oesophageal intubation
- Tracheal tube in right main bronchus
- Kinked tracheal tube
- Tracheal tube cuff herniation over end of tube
- Secretions in tracheal tube
- Secretions in trachea/lungs
- Gastric acid aspiration
- Pneumothorax
- Pulmonary oedema
- Bronchospasm

Complications associated with intubation often cause wheeze, and it is essential to check the position and patency of the tracheal tube first.

Treatment

Treatment of intraoperative bronchospasm is as follows:
1 Consider using a volatile agent.
2 Give salbutamol 250 μg slowly intravenously.

3 Give aminophylline 250–500 mg (4–8 mg/kg) intravenously over 10–15 minutes.
4 Give adrenaline (epinephrine) 0.5–1.0 ml 1 : 10,000 increments intravenously.
5 Give hydrocortisone 100 mg intravenously.

18.3 Aspiration

Several factors make patients more prone to vomiting and aspiration of gastric contents in anaesthesia. These include trauma, a full stomach, opioids, raised gastric pressure (bowel obstruction, pregnancy) and diabetes. Aspiration may be particulate or liquid and concealed or obvious. Use of an appropriate anaesthetic technique (i.e. rapid sequence induction) safeguards patients most at risk.

Patients with wheeze must be suspected of having aspirated, and a postoperative chest x-ray may reveal a right lobe infiltrative pattern. Aspiration usually occurs into the right lung.

Treatment

Treatment is aimed at securing the airway, aspirating the trachea and ensuring oxygenation. If aspiration is severe, surgery should be abandoned. Saline lavage of the trachea and bronchi may be useful (under supervision), antibiotics are given, and steroids are often used. The patient must be monitored closely postoperatively.

18.4 Cyanosis

See Chapter 19, Section 19.7.

18.5 Arrhythmias

Arrhythmias often occur in healthy patients undergoing anaesthesia. It is often difficult to interpret the ECG trace with only 6–7 beats observed on the screen. Atrial and ventricular ectopic beats are usually easily identified, but changes in P waves and ST segment changes may be hard to discern until extreme. Many modern monitors perform ST segment analysis routinely. Electrolyte abnormalities, especially hypokalaemia and hypomagnesaemia, should be treated.

Treatment

If any anaesthetic or surgical cause for the arrhythmia is eliminated and the rhythm disturbance remains, then five courses of action should be considered:

1 observation + no treatment
2 physical intervention
3 drug treatment
4 cardioversion
5 pacing

Careful observation with no immediate treatment is commonly undertaken in patients with occasional atrial and ventricular ectopic beats who are cardiovascularly stable (normal blood pressure and no evidence of cardiac failure). Physical interventions, other than the removal of retractors that may compress the heart, consist of stopping the surgery when a vagal response, such as a severe bradycardia or even a brief asystolic episode, occurs. Arrhythmias are often transient, but they can age the novice anaesthetist – who will, briefly, wish for a career in dermatology! Carotid sinus massage and gentle pressure on the eye are ineffective treatments for supraventricular tachycardias found under anaesthesia. Careful preoperative assessment should identify those patients who may need pacing, and it is very unusual to need intraoperative pacing (complete heart block or symptomatic heart block). The drug treatments of life-threatening arrhythmias that we have found useful are summarised in Box 18.4. It is difficult to distinguish narrow and broad complex tachycardias during anaesthesia. A 12-lead electrocardiograph is needed, and this is often impractical during surgery.

Box 18.4 Drug treatment of life-threatening arrhythmias

- Sinus bradycardia
  - atropine 0.3 mg increments
- Narrow complex tachycardias
  - adenosine 6 mg rapid bolus followed by second dose of 12 mg within 1 minute, if necessary
  - if hypotensive, signs of failure and heart rate more than 200, give amiodarone 300 mg slowly and consider electrical cardioversion
- Broad complex tachycardias (pulse present)
  - amiodarone 150 mg over 10 minutes
    or
  - lignocaine (lidocaine) 50 mg over 5 minutes (repeated × 3)
- Sudden-onset atrial fibrillation
  - amiodarone 300 mg slowly

For the tachyarrhythmias listed in Box 18.4, synchronised DC cardioversion must be considered if there are signs of heart failure, if blood pressure is less than 90 mm Hg, or if there is a sustained heart rate of more than 150/minute

18.6 Hypotension

Intraoperative hypotension is common and usually results from an inadequate blood volume following haemorrhage. The major causes are either a decreased venous return or a direct depression of the myocardium due to mechanical causes, myocardial disease or anaesthetic drugs (Box 18.5).

Box 18.5 Major causes of intraoperative hypotension

- Decreased venous return
  - haemorrhage
  - vena caval compression – obstetrics, prone position
  - drugs, infection
  - anaesthesia without surgery
  - anaphylaxis
  - sepsis
  - epidural analgesia
- Myocardial depression
  - mechanical
  - intermittent positive pressure ventilation
    - equipment and circuit malfunction
    - pneumothorax
    - cardiac tamponade
    - pulmonary embolus
  - cardiac disease
  - drugs

Treatment

Treatment is dependent on correct identification of the cause. Rapid intravenous infusion of colloid or blood may be required, together with measurement of the central venous pressure. The use of inotropic drugs should be considered only when you are sure that there is an adequate circulating blood volume. Adrenaline is not an appropriate treatment for the hypotension of haemorrhage. Ensure that the hypotension is not a measurement error. Also check that there is not an excessive concentration of volatile agent.

18.7 Hypertension

Hypertension can occur from many causes, and these are listed in Box 18.6.

Box 18.6 Causes of intraoperative hypertension

- Sympathetic stimulation
  - hypoxia, hypercarbia
  - inadequate level of anaesthesia, awareness
  - pain
  - raised intracranial pressure
- Iatrogenic
  - incorrect drug administration
- Rare causes
  - malignant hyperthermia
  - phaeochromocytoma

Treatment

Treatment is based on finding the cause of hypertension. Lack of analgesia or anaesthesia are the commonest causes. Ensure that the measurement is correct before starting treatment.

18.8 Conclusion

Many problems occur during the induction and maintenance of anaesthesia, and during recovery of a patient. Whatever the problem, a cause must be sought in the following sequence: anaesthetic > surgical > medical. Only when the first two have been eliminated should specific medical therapy be started.

Chapter 19 **Postoperative problems**

Intraoperative problems described in the previous chapter (laryngospasm, wheeze, aspiration, cyanosis, arrhythmias, hypotension, hypertension) may continue, or even start, in the postoperative period. Investigation of the cause and subsequent management of these problems is identical, regardless of the time of onset.

19.1 Airway obstruction

Obstruction of the airway is a common occurrence after anaesthesia. It must be rapidly diagnosed (Box 19.1), the cause sought (Box 19.2), and appropriate treatment started.

Box 19.1 Signs of airway obstruction

- 'See-saw' respiration pattern
- Suprasternal and intercostal recession
- Tachypnoea
- Cyanosis
- Tachycardia
- Arrhythmias
- Hypertension
- Anxiety and distress
- Sweating
- Stridor

How to Survive in Anaesthesia: A Guide for Trainees, Fourth Edition.
Neville Robinson, George Hall and William Fawcett.
© 2012 John Wiley & Sons, Ltd. Published 2012 by John Wiley & Sons, Ltd.

Box 19.2 Common causes of postoperative airway obstruction

- Anaesthesia
  - unconsciousness with obstruction by tongue
  - pharyngeal muscle weakness
  - laryngeal oedema
  - laryngospasm (Chapter 18)
- Surgery
  - vocal cord paralysis (thyroid surgery)
  - neck haematoma
  - preoperative neck and face inflammation (infection)

During emergence from anaesthesia patients may have pharyngeal and laryngeal muscle weakness, causing airway obstruction. Hypoxaemia will result if the airway is not maintained. Patients are turned routinely into the lateral or 'recovery position' to help prevent this problem. The patient is usually placed in the left lateral position, as reintubation is easier because laryngoscopes are designed to be inserted into the right side of the mouth. Curiously, most anaesthetists sleep in the recovery position.

If there is a possibility that aspiration may have occurred with the patient in the supine position, then he or she should be placed in the right lateral position to prevent contamination of the left lung.

Patients who are at risk of aspiration should be extubated when the airway reflexes are intact. Although this is less pleasant for the patient, it is much safer.

The treatment of airway obstruction is to identify the cause, and clear the airway, often with suction, to ensure patency. Extension of the neck, jaw thrust, and insertion of an oropharyngeal airway are often required. Laryngeal oedema is treated by intravenous dexamethasone 8 mg. Oxygenation of the patient is the priority, and, if you are in doubt, reintubation must be undertaken. Many problems in anaesthesia are caused by inadequate attention to the airway. Remember, a patent airway is a happy airway.

19.2 Failure to breathe

Failure to breathe adequately at the end of anaesthesia has many causes, both common (Box 19.3) and unusual (Box 19.4).

Box 19.3 Common causes of failure to breathe

- Central nervous system
  - depression from drugs
    - opioids
    - inhalational agents
  - decreased respiratory drive
    - hypocapnia
- Peripheral nervous system
  - failure of neuromuscular transmission
    - inadequate reversal of competitive relaxants
    - overdosage of competitive relaxants
    - pseudocholinesterase deficiency

Box 19.4 Unusual causes of failure to breathe

- Hypothermia
- Drug interactions
  - aminoglycosides and competitive relaxants
  - ecothiopate and suxamethonium
- Central nervous system damage
- Electrolyte disorders
  - hypokalaemia
- Undiagnosed skeletal muscle disorders
  - myasthenia gravis
- Extensive spinal anaesthetic in combination with general anaesthesia

Differentiation between central and peripheral causes of failure to breathe can only be made by using a nerve stimulator. A peripheral nerve, such as the ulnar nerve at the wrist, is stimulated. Ensure that the nerve stimulator is working correctly – if necessary, try it on yourself first.

Adequate return of neuromuscular function is assessed by observing a 'train of four' stimulation. Four twitches should be seen and the ratio of twitch 4 : twitch 1 response must exceed 70%. This is not easy to decide, and we recommend that they should appear about equal. This ensures safety. A sustained tetanic response following high-frequency stimulation also indicates adequate neuromuscular function (Box 19.5).

Box 19.5 Signs of adequate neuromuscular function

- Clinical responses
  - lift head for 5 seconds
  - sustained hand grip
  - effective cough
  - adequate tidal volume
  - vital capacity 15–20 ml/kg
- Evoked responses
  - train-of-four ratio should appear equal
  - sustained tetanic response to high-frequency stimulation
  - return of single twitch to control height

If a nerve stimulator is not available, there are clinical tests that can be made to indicate the return of normal neuromuscular activity. If inadequate neuromuscular function is found, the lungs must be ventilated and the use of neuromuscular blocking drugs reviewed.

Prolonged apnoea after suxamethonium occurs when the patient has an abnormal genetic variant of the plasma enzyme pseudocholinesterase. The patient and members of the family should be investigated at a later date, and susceptible individuals asked to carry warning cards.

Only when you are certain that neuromuscular transmission is normal should a central cause for failure to breathe be considered. Again the lungs must be ventilated, a normal end-tidal CO_2 concentration obtained and possible causes assessed (Box 19.3).

An overdose of opioid is a common reason for failure to breathe. This can be treated with low doses of intravenous naloxone 40 µg, but this potent antagonist is short-acting and the return of adequate respiration is usually accompanied by a complete lack of analgesia! This is an unsatisfactory mess and it is better to ventilate the lungs until the central depressant effects of the drugs have worn off, or consider intravenous doxapram. A new drug, sugammadex, can rapidly reverse the muscle relaxation caused by rocuronium and vecuronium.

19.3 Nausea and vomiting

Nausea and vomiting are particularly unpleasant complications of anaesthesia and surgery. The avoidance of these problems is more important to some patients than the provision of adequate analgesia. There are many factors associated with the occurrence of nausea and vomiting (Box 19.6). This long list indicates that often there is no single identifiable cause, although opioids are frequently at fault.

Box 19.6 Factors associated with postoperative vomiting

- Patient predisposition
  - age, sex, menstrual cycle, obesity
  - history of postoperative vomiting
  - history of motion sickness
  - anxiety, pain
  - recent food intake, prolonged fasting
- Surgical factors
  - type of surgery, e.g. squint repair and laparoscopic surgery
  - emergency surgery
- Anaesthetic factors
  - inhalational agents and nitrous oxide
  - opioids
  - duration of anaesthesia
  - distension of gut
  - oropharyngeal stimulation
  - experience of anaesthetist
- Postoperative factors
  - pain
  - hypotension
  - hypoxaemia
  - movement of patient
  - first intake of fluids/food
  - early mobilisation

Because patients find nausea and vomiting distressing, it should be prevented if possible. The medical consequences of vomiting include the possibility of acid aspiration, electrolyte imbalance and dehydration, inability to take oral drugs and disruption of the wound. A vomiting patient also upsets other patients in the recovery area and surgical ward.

Most anaesthetists prescribe antiemetics, but the consensus is that they should not be given prophylactically unless patients are deemed high risk. Drugs used include cyclizine, prochlorperazine, droperidol, metoclopramide, dexamethasone and ondansetron. A combination of antiemetics is often required.

19.4 Delayed awakening

Failure to recover full consciousness after surgery is always worrying for the anaesthetist. A systematic review of the patient is necessary (Box 19.7).

Box 19.7 Causes of delayed recovery

- Hypoxaemia
- Hypercapnia
- Residual anaesthesia
- Drugs, especially opioids
- Emergence delirium from ketamine, scopolamine, atropine
- Neurological causes
- Surgery: neurosurgery, vascular surgery
- Metabolic causes
  - hypoglycaemia
  - hyponatraemia
- Medical causes
  - hypothyroidism
- Sepsis
- Hypothermia

The most common causes are drug-related, but you must also remember the possibility of a low temperature, low blood glucose, low plasma sodium and low circulating thyroid hormones.

19.5 Shivering

Shivering is common during recovery from anaesthesia, but is not obviously related to a low core temperature in the patient. It is more frequent in young men who have received volatile agents, and its incidence is decreased by the use of opioids during anaesthesia. The main deleterious effect of shivering is an increase in O_2 consumption. This is of little consequence in young, fit patients, but it should be treated promptly in the elderly, who often have impaired cardiac and respiratory function.

Pethidine 25 mg intravenously is effective in stopping shivering; other opioids can also be used. Low doses of intravenous doxapram are an alternative to opioids if there is a risk of respiratory depression. The simple application of heat to the 'blush area' (the face and upper chest) stops shivering. This indicates the importance of skin temperature in stimulating shivering, as the effect on body temperature is negligible.

19.6 Temperature disturbances

A decrease in body temperature is an inevitable accompaniment of anaesthesia. Indeed, it has been noted that the most effective means of cooling a person is to give an anaesthetic. Hypothermia (defined as a core temperature less than 35 °C) can occur after major surgery, and the predisposing factors are shown in Box 19.8.

Box 19.8 Factors predisposing to postoperative hypothermia

• Ambient theatre temperature
• Age: young and elderly
• Surgery
  – duration
  – size of incision
  – insulation
• Concomitant disease
• Intravenous fluid administration
• Drug therapy such as vasodilators

Complications of postoperative hypothermia may include shivering (see above), impaired drug metabolism and decreased platelet aggregation. There are several methods available for preventing loss of body heat during surgery (Box 19.9), and a combination of treatments is necessary. For example, the theatre temperature must be maintained at 24 °C, the inspired gases humidified, the intravenous fluids warmed and the skin surface warmed.

Box 19.9 Prevention of body heat loss

• Ambient theatre temperature
• Airway humidification
• Warm skin surface
  – passive insulation
  – active warming
    • water blanket

- radiant heater
- forced air warmer
- Warm intravenous fluids

Hyperthermia after anaesthesia is uncommon. Of the causes listed in Box 19.10, infection is the most common, and the potentially lethal complication of malignant hyperthermia should be diagnosed only after arterial gas analysis and determination of circulating potassium values (see Chapter 14).

Box 19.10 Causes of hyperthermia

- Infection
- Environmental
- Mismatched transfusion
- Drugs
    - interactions
    - atropine overdose
- Metabolic
    - malignant hyperthermia
    - phaeochromocytoma
    - hyperthyroidism

19.7 Cyanosis

Cyanosis is a serious sequela of anaesthesia and, whenever it occurs, must be investigated promptly.
1 Check for patent airway. If intubated, is tracheal tube correctly positioned and patent?
2 Check oxygen delivery from anaesthetic circuit.
3 Having excluded these causes, consider:
    fault in chest (is ventilation easy?)
    - bronchospasm
    - pulmonary oedema
    - pneumothorax
    - pleural effusion/haemothorax
    fault in circulation
    - decreased venous return
    - cardiac failure
    - embolism
    - drug reaction

4 Rare causes include:
- methaemoglobinaemia
- malignant hyperthermia

Problems of the airway are the most common causes of cyanosis, and you must be *certain* that the airway is patent and the patient is breathing O_2 before considering other causes. Unless the situation is rapidly diagnosed and corrected the patient will need urgent tracheal intubation, ventilation with 100% oxygen, and resuscitation along conventional guidelines. Remember pneumothorax and cardiac tamponade, especially if the patient has undergone central line insertion. Both require specific (and life-saving) therapy. In cases associated with circulatory changes, fluids and/or sympathomimetics may be required.

19.8 Conclusion

Postoperative problems often reflect errors of judgement made during surgery. Get it right intraoperatively and your patients will have fewer difficulties postoperatively. Nursing staff in the recovery area and surgical wards rapidly assess your anaesthetic skills by the smoothness of recovery of your patients.

Chapter 20 **Anaesthetic mishaps**

In previous chapters we have described the management of problems that a trainee anaesthetist would be expected to recognise and treat. Unfortunately, errors made by the anaesthetist also result in morbidity and occasionally even mortality.

We give examples below of common mistakes made by anaesthetists, young and old, that we have seen in recent years.

20.1 Intravenous cannulae and infusions

Ensure that the intravenous cannula is in the vein! Although this states the obvious, we keep seeing examples of cannulae that are subcutaneous and even in the dressing. If the patient arrives in the operating theatre with an intravenous cannula in place, remove all the dressings, examine it carefully and check for patency by flushing with 0.9% sodium chloride solution. If in doubt, insert another cannula. The cannula for total intravenous anaesthesia (TIVA) must be in a vein. Total subcutaneous anaesthesia is not effective and the patient will be aware! Always ensure that you have easy access to the giving set for drug administration. Arms by the side can cause problems.

When inserting a cannula, do not place the introducing needle on the patient or trolley. A needle-stick injury to the anaesthetic, theatre, recovery or ward staff will ensure that you are omitted from all future social events.

Anaesthetists often have two speeds for intravenous infusions: off and full open. The 'full open' infusion is a problem if additions have been made to the infusion fluid. The rapid infusion of 20–40 mmol potassium is bad for the health of both patient and anaesthetist.

How to Survive in Anaesthesia: A Guide for Trainees, Fourth Edition.
Neville Robinson, George Hall and William Fawcett.
© 2012 John Wiley & Sons, Ltd. Published 2012 by John Wiley & Sons, Ltd.

20.2 Drugs

All syringes must be labelled correctly. For example, recently a 2 ml syringe containing suxamethonium was labelled incorrectly as antiemetic. Patients do not expect to have nausea and vomiting treated by the rapid onset of paralysis.

Atropine and adrenaline are often stored next to each in the drug cupboard, and the wrong drug has been drawn up by an inexperienced assistant in an emergency.

It is easy to forget to add the drug to the solvent. One author has, on two occasions, failed to add the vecuronium to the diluent and waited for the onset of paralysis for many minutes.

Emergency drugs, suxamethonium and atropine, should be checked and drawn up at the beginning of the list. It is easy to assume that they are readily available. One author had the alarming experience of a patient suddenly developing severe sinus bradycardia from direct vagal stimulation (less than 30 beats/minute) with no atropine available in the theatres. Fortunately, the patient survived – but the mistake has never been repeated.

20.3 Anaesthetic machine and equipment

It is important to remember that with machines and equipment, if anything can go wrong, it will go wrong. You are surrounded in life by examples of technical failures. They will follow you into the operating theatre.

Anaesthetic tubing invariably becomes disconnected at the most inconvenient time. The oxygen flush device can stick on, which is noisy and embarrassing. Modern anaesthetic machines can be fraught with problems. For example, after each case the machine can reset and return to air and not nitrous oxide so that the patient is at risk from awareness. Some ventilators require the 'on' switch to be held down for a few seconds to start. In the circle system there is often a switch for spontaneous ventilation and controlled ventilation. Always keep a self-inflating bag on the machine so you can use this when all else fails.

Vaporisers are often the source of problems. They may not have been filled at the start of the list, or they may not be seated correctly on the back bar of the anaesthetic machine, with a consequent leak of gases. These errors are common if the vaporiser is changed during an anaesthetic.

Ensure that all ancillary equipment functions correctly. The failure to have spare laryngoscopes with bulbs that work and the failure to replace suction equipment after use have resulted in the unnecessary deaths of patients. Checking the equipment is your responsibility.

20.4 Monitoring equipment

Monitoring equipment fails occasionally, and can also display misleading values. A spare set of monitoring equipment must always be available. Always support the information given by the monitors with direct observation of the patient. Assume that the monitoring will fail at the most inappropriate time. One author had a complete failure of all intravascular pressure measurements during anaesthesia for a phaeochromocytoma.

Some anaesthetists disable the alarms on the monitor. This is stupidity. Ensure that alarms are on and set within sensible limits. With gas analysis and MAC displayed, you will know that your patient is breathing correct quantities of oxygen and is properly anaesthetised. Remember not to rely on pulse oximetry unless you have a good plethysmograph trace – we have seen good SpO_2 readings with the probe on the pillow.

20.5 Tracheal tubes

Very occasionally you will be certain that you saw the tube pass between the vocal cords into the trachea and yet you have inserted the tube into the oesophagus. Because you are sure that the tube is in the correct place, you try to explain the failure to ventilate the lungs as a problem with the patient, for example bronchospasm. We know of at least four occasions on which this error has occurred. If the mistake is not rectified the patient will die. If in doubt, remove the tube, ventilate the patient and reinsert the tube correctly. Tracheal tubes can also be inserted too far, kink and become obstructed.

20.6 Epidural anaesthesia

Epidural catheter sets can have manufacturing faults. The most common is the absence of holes in the end of the epidural catheter so that it is impossible to inject drugs. Many drugs have been given in error through the epidural catheter. Antibiotics and thiopentone are particular favourites, as they are usually in a 20 ml syringe, the same volume as the local anaesthetic. Be particularly careful when the epidural catheter and filter are placed next to the central venous cannula. Conversely, local anaesthetic solutions have been given intravenously in error, causing convulsions and even death.

20.7 Transfer of patients

Ensure that the patient is adequately anaesthetised before transfer from the anaesthetic room into theatre. Failure to do so results in a shambles. One author recently had the patient sit up in theatre, remove the laryngeal mask and hand it to the surgeon! Try to avoid being the cabaret act in theatre.

Similarly, transfer to the recovery area at the end of surgery can also degenerate into chaos. A violent patient with an obstructed airway is not easy to sort out in the corridor. Stay in theatre until you are sure that the patient is safe.

20.8 Theatre environment

There are many distractions in theatre. Keep all unnecessary people out of the anaesthetic room. It should not be used as a venue for social intercourse – the nocturnal habits of Sharon and Darren may be interesting but will divert your concentration away from the patient. Music in the theatre may interfere with hearing of the alarms on the anaesthetic machine or monitoring equipment. If so, the music must be turned down or off.

20.9 Conclusion

Get used to continually checking and re-checking the patient and monitors. Ensure you have good access to the patient's airway and intravenous cannula. Pay particular attention to the expired CO_2, SpO_2, ECG, blood pressure and MAC values. Never be frightened to share your concerns with theatre staff – all will rally to your support. Anaesthesia has the uncanny habit of humbling overconfident, arrogant anaesthetists who believe that they never make mistakes.

Unfortunately, simple mistakes can kill patients.

Part III **Passing the gas**

As the weeks of your anaesthetic career become months, you will play a larger role in the preoperative assessment of patients and the conduct of the anaesthetic.

In this section of the book we describe briefly the anaesthetic considerations of some of the common surgical specialties with which a trainee is often involved. We have deliberately excluded any pharmacology of the anaesthetic drugs; trainees should obtain an appropriate pharmacology textbook. There is no evidence to show any benefit from a particular anaesthetic technique in terms of postoperative morbidity and mortality. The principles of anaesthesia are more important than the choice of drugs.

The key feature of this section is the need for a thorough preoperative evaluation of all patients. This is the cornerstone of safe anaesthetic practice and must *never* be omitted.

Chapter 21 **Preoperative evaluation**

Preoperative evaluation is used to assess the anaesthetic risks in relation to the proposed surgery, to decide the anaesthetic technique (general, regional, or a combination) and to plan the postoperative care, including any analgesic regimens. Explanation of the relevant details of the anaesthetic can be given. Patients waiting for surgery are vulnerable, and therefore a friendly, professional approach by the anaesthetist is essential.

Operations are classified into four groups that define the urgency of the surgery (Box 21.1). This classification has been agreed with the surgeons, but their memory often fails, so do not be surprised to find elective cases suddenly classified as emergencies! This is usually done for surgical convenience.

Box 21.1 Classification of operations

- Immediate   Immediate life-, limb- or organ-saving intervention – resuscitation simultaneous with intervention. Normally within minutes of decision to operate. (A) life-saving; (B) other, e.g. limb- or organ-saving
- Urgent   Intervention in response to acute onset or clinical deterioration of potentially life-threatening conditions, for those conditions that may threaten the survival of limb or organ, for fixation of many fractures and for relief of pain or other distressing symptoms. Normally within hours of decision to operate
- Expedited   Patient requiring early treatment where the condition is not an immediate threat to life, limb or organ survival. Normally within days of decision to operate
- Elective   Intervention planned or booked in advance of routine admission to hospital. Timing to suit patient, hospital and staff

---

How to Survive in Anaesthesia: A Guide for Trainees, Fourth Edition.
Neville Robinson, George Hall and William Fawcett.
© 2012 John Wiley & Sons, Ltd. Published 2012 by John Wiley & Sons, Ltd.

It is sometimes difficult to convey an overall impression of the complexity of a patient's medical condition, and this can be done by referring to one of the five American Society of Anesthesiologists (ASA) physical status classes (Box 21.2). It is important to remember that this only refers to the physical status of the patient and does not consider other relevant factors such as age, and nature and duration of surgery.

Box 21.2 ASA physical status classes

- ASA 1   normal healthy patient
- ASA 2   patient with mild controlled systemic disease that does not affect normal activity, e.g. mild diabetes, mild hypertension
- ASA 3   patient with severe systemic disease which limits activity, e.g. angina, chronic bronchitis
- ASA 4   patient with incapacitating systemic disease that is a constant threat to life
- ASA 5   moribund patient not expected to survive 24 hours either with or without an operation
- E   emergency procedure

Preoperative assessment is outlined below:

1 history
- age
- present illness
- drugs
- allergies
- past history (operations and anaesthetics)
- anaesthetic family history
- social (smoking, alcohol)

2 examination
- AIRWAY (see Chapter 1)
- teeth
- general examination

3 specific assessment
4 investigations
5 consent
6 premedication, if required

The history of the present illness is important. For example, in orthopaedic surgery, a fractured neck of femur may occur for many reasons: a fall from an accident, stroke, cardiac episode (Stokes–Adams attack) or a spontaneous fracture from a metastasis.

The subsequent examination and investigations are obviously different in each case. Details of any previous anaesthetics may indicate difficulties with tracheal intubation. Unfortunately, successful intubation in the past is no guarantee of future success. A family history of pseudocholinesterase deficiency and malignant hyperthermia should be sought.

A specific assessment of the concurrent disease(s) must also be undertaken. The problem of obesity (BMI > 30) is evaluated as shown in Box 21.3.

Box 21.3 Specific assessment of obesity

- Psychological aspects
- Drug metabolism
- Associated diseases
  - hypertension
  - coronary artery disease
  - diabetes
- Difficult venous access
- Airway
  - difficult to intubate
  - difficult to maintain
  - reflux
- Hypoxaemia more likely intraoperatively – ventilation mandatory
- Regional anaesthesia – difficult to perform
- Position of patient for surgery
- Blood pressure measurements difficult (cuff size)
- Postoperative analgesia and physiotherapy to decrease chest complications
- Immobility and deep vein thrombosis – prophylaxis
- Wound dehiscence and wound infection

Only appropriate investigations should be undertaken. A typical list of basic tests is shown in Box 21.4.

Box 21.4 Basic and advanced preoperative tests

- Basic
  - haemoglobin concentration
  - screening for sickle cell disease

> - blood urea, creatinine and electrolyte concentrations
> - blood glucose
> - chest x-ray film
> - ECG
> • Advanced
>   - respiratory function tests
>   - echocardiography
>   - arterial blood gases
>   - clotting profile
>   - cardiopulmonary exercise testing

A lot of money is wasted on unnecessary preoperative tests. When you have taken a history from the patient and conducted the relevant examination, you must then decide what tests, if any, are required. A young, fit sportsman for an arthroscopy requires no further investigation. An elderly West Indian patient who has diabetes, hypertension, coronary artery disease, and needs major vascular surgery, requires all the basic tests listed in Box 21.4 and probably more. In many hospitals there are guidelines on the use of preoperative investigations. These can be helpful, as they reflect local practice. For example, you may find that there is far greater use of preoperative chest x-ray films in regions with a high population of recent immigrants, to exclude tuberculosis.

On completion of the preoperative assessment, and with the results of the relevant investigations available, a plan for the anaesthetic care of the patient can be decided. The following surgical factors must also be considered:
• When is the operation to occur?
• Who is operating?
• Where is the patient going postoperatively (home, ward, HDU, ICU)?
Occasionally, it is necessary to postpone surgery. This is most often done on medical grounds, for example to improve cardiac failure, treat arrhythmias and control blood pressure. In the early months of your anaesthetic career, seek senior advice before postponing surgery – this prevents prolonged arguments with surgical colleagues.

21.1 Premedication

The use of premedication is declining, although most anaesthetists undergoing surgery demand heavy sedation. The wishes of the patient must be considered. The main reasons for giving premedication are shown in Box 21.5.

> **Box 21.5** Reasons for premedication
>
> - Anxiolysis
> - Antisialagogue
> - Analgesia
> - Antiemesis
> - Amnesia
> - Decreased gastric acidity
> - Part of anaesthetic technique (assist induction)
> - Prevention of unwanted vagal responses
> - Prevention of needle pain

A variety of drugs including opioids, benzodiazepines, anticholinergics, phenothiazines and H_2 receptor blocking drugs are used. It is important to remember that opioids may make patients vomit. Topical EMLA cream can be used to prevent the pain of insertion of a cannula. This eutectic mixture of prilocaine and lignocaine (1 g of EMLA contains 25 mg of each) is applied to the dorsum of the hands for a minimum of 1 hour to a maximum of 5 hours before induction of anaesthesia.

21.2 Drug therapy

Drug therapy is usually continued throughout the operative period, especially cardiac and antihypertensive drugs. Notable exceptions are the hypoglycaemic drugs and clopidogrel. Patients taking oral contraceptives and hormone replacement therapy require thromboprophylaxis with subcutaneous low-molecular-weight heparin and graduated elastic compression stockings. Potential interactions with anaesthetic drugs should be considered.

21.3 Preoperative starvation

An empty stomach decreases the risk of vomiting and regurgitation. Food is usually withheld for 6 hours before elective surgery and in some hospitals it is now common practice to allow clear fluids until 2 hours before surgery. For emergency surgery these guidelines are inappropriate, and the only safe practice is to assume that the stomach is not empty (see Chapter 23).

21.4 When to ask for advice

A common difficulty for the trainee is when to ask for advice and assistance. We suggest that if you need advice, state that you are ringing for advice. If you need a senior member of the team to be present you should say so.

If in doubt, it is always better to inform seniors of the problems and your decisions. Often two minds are better than one, and senior anaesthetists need to know what is happening in the department, especially out of routine working hours.

21.5 Conclusion

Preoperative assessment is often difficult, and its importance should not be underestimated. The anaesthetic care of the patient can only be planned after a thorough assessment, together with the results of relevant investigations, and precise knowledge of the proposed surgery. In emergency surgery, ask the question 'Can the patient be made significantly better? If so, does time allow this?'

Chapter 22 **Recognition and management of the sick patient**

The anaesthetic trainee is often called to a ward to assess and initiate treatment of the ill patient. The correct diagnosis must be established, resuscitation started and the patient stabilised.

A patient who requires emergency surgery should ideally have full resuscitation and stabilisation before surgery. However, a balance needs to be struck between the benefits of restoring physiological normality and the dangers of delaying surgery. Often this judgement requires senior help.

Principles of care are outlined in Box 22.1.

Box 22.1 Principles of care in the sick surgical patient

- Correct diagnosis – team approach
- Where to resuscitate
- Communication
  - address individuals
  - be heard
  - be understood
- Notify operating theatre and relevant staff
- Treat patient
  - oxygen therapy
  - intravenous fluids
    - urinary catheter
    - cardiovascular – invasive or non-invasive monitoring
    - gastric stasis – nasogastric tube (trauma, sepsis, diabetes)
    - analgesia
    - drugs – antibiotics, inotropes, diuretics
- Transfer of patient

How to Survive in Anaesthesia: A Guide for Trainees, Fourth Edition.
Neville Robinson, George Hall and William Fawcett.
© 2012 John Wiley & Sons, Ltd. Published 2012 by John Wiley & Sons, Ltd.

Sick patients are often in cubicles with other patients. Anything you say may be overheard, so avoid criticisms of care and insinuations of blame. Be professional and discreet.

Ward patients are observed and their recordings are subject to a trigger scoring system (Early Warning Scores, or EWS). The heart rate, temperature, blood pressure and urine output are monitored. Normal recordings score 0 but abnormally high or low recordings score up to 3. The scores are added, and when the sum exceeds a nominated theshold (normally 3) medical assessment of the patient should occur.

22.1 Diagnosis

Do not assume that the diagnosis given by the ward staff is correct. Hypotension and tachycardia after surgery are more likely to result from hypovolaemia and haemorrhage than myocardial infarction. Similarly, an unconscious patient may have suffered a stroke, but other causes must be sought (see Box 19.7). Examine the patient yourself to confirm or refute the tentative diagnosis. A heart rate over 100/minute is abnormal!

22.2 Where to resuscitate

Wards often have poor lighting, few staff at night, and the drugs and equipment needed are usually unavailable. Attempts to resuscitate the patient in such surroundings almost inevitably waste time, and it is much easier to transfer the patient to a place where staff are familiar with invasive procedures. Suitable environments are the theatre recovery area, an anaesthetic room and the high dependency unit. If the patient is in the accident and emergency unit, it is usually safer to manage them there until stable.

22.3 Communication

Two situations commonly occur. First, you are left with no staff to help, and second, there are many people available and yet nothing is happening. In the first instance, get help; one knowledgeable and skilled assistant is ideal. In the second situation, take charge. When you want something to be done, address specific people, speak clearly and ensure you are heard and understood. Insist that the person reports back when the instruction has been fulfilled. Record events clearly, although this may have to be done later. If the patient needs to go to theatre urgently, inform theatre staff.

22.4 Treatment

Oxygenation is a priority. A suitable mask should be placed on the patient's face and the oxygen supply turned on. Wards often only have variable performance masks available, and an oxygen flow rate of 6 litres/minute is necessary to increase the inspired oxygen to about 50%.

Intravenous fluids should be given. Either 0.9% sodium chloride solution or Hartmann's solution are the fluids of choice if a crystalloid is required. Colloids may be necessary if there is obvious haemorrhage (see Chapter 6, Tables 6.1 and 6.2).

Appropriate monitoring should be established. If necessary, direct measurement of arterial pressure and central venous pressure should be undertaken (see Chapter 5). Fluid replacement is then guided by these intravascular pressures. Initially, a systolic arterial pressure of more than 100 mm Hg usually ensures that perfusion of the key organs is adequate. The adequacy of renal perfusion is often assessed by measuring urine output. A urinary catheter is essential for accurate measurement, and the output should be more than 0.5 ml/kg/h. Inotropic support may be required if an arterial pressure cannot be achieved after optimal filling of the circulation.

Gastric stasis can develop rapidly in sick patients, and it may be necessary to insert a nasogastric tube.

Analgesia may be required. Small bolus intravenous injections of morphine 1–2 mg are the safest method of achieving pain relief in sick patients.

An adequately resuscitated patient will have:
- heart rate < 80/min
- respiratory rate < 18/min
- systolic pressure > 100 mm Hg
- CVP > 5 mm Hg and no increase on fluid challenge
- urine output > 0.5 ml/kg/h
- ABG base excess below –3 mmol/l
- blood lactate < 1.5 mmol/l

22.5 Transfer of patients

Sick patients go on journeys round hospitals, and these trips are potentially dangerous. The patient must only be moved when suitable members of staff are available with appropriate monitoring. It is unacceptable to resuscitate a sick patient with full monitoring and then remove most of it for transfer. When moving the patient, guard carefully venous and arterial cannulae, catheters, drips, drains etc. so that they are not pulled out.

Be certain that staff will be available to help on arrival – this is a particular problem in radiology departments at night.

22.6 Conclusion

Rescuing sick patients from wards often falls to trainee anaesthetists because of their knowledge of resuscitation and technical skills. If in doubt, move the patient to a place where you have the necessary skilled staff, drugs and equipment.

Chapter 23 **Principles of emergency anaesthesia**

In elective surgery the correct diagnosis has been made (usually), any medical disorders have been identified and treated, and an appropriate period of starvation has been determined. During emergency work, however, one or more of these conditions are often not met. In addition, there are further problems such as:

- dehydration
- electrolyte abnormalities
- haemorrhage
- pain

The components of general anaesthesia are the same, whether it is conducted for elective surgery or emergency surgery (Box 23.1).

Box 23.1 Components of general anaesthesia

- Preoperative assessment
- Premedication, if any
- Induction
- Maintenance
- Reversal
- Postoperative care

The key to success in emergency anaesthesia is a thorough preoperative assessment. It should be undertaken as described in Chapter 21. Particular attention must be given to medical problems, the occurrence of hypovolaemia and an evaluation of the airway. On the basis of the preoperative clinical

How to Survive in Anaesthesia: A Guide for Trainees, Fourth Edition.
Neville Robinson, George Hall and William Fawcett.
© 2012 John Wiley & Sons, Ltd. Published 2012 by John Wiley & Sons, Ltd.

assessment, together with the results of *relevant* investigations, a decision for an appropriate time to operate can be reached.

There are very few patients with a potentially life-threatening clinical state that need immediate surgery, i.e. a true 'emergency' (see Box 21.1). A vast majority of patients greatly benefit from the correction of hypovolaemia and electrolyte abnormalities, stabilisation of medical problems, such as diabetes and cardiac arrhythmias, and waiting for the stomach to empty.

If necessary, preoperative optimisation should be undertaken in ICU. Surgeons are not known for their patience and often view any delay in operating as time wasted. *When to operate* is the most important decision that has to be made in emergency work. Fortunately, for the patient, and for you, increasingly this decision is made by senior staff. In the early stages of your anaesthetic career you should observe closely the evidence used to reach such a decision.

Although it is usually assumed that emergency anaesthesia means general anaesthesia, other methods can sometimes be employed (Box 23.2).

Box 23.2 Classification of anaesthetic techniques

- General anaesthesia
  - intubation of unprotected airway
  - spontaneous respiration or controlled ventilation
  - use of muscle relaxants
- Regional anaesthesia
- Combination of general and regional anaesthesia
- Sedation
  - intravenous
  - inhalational
- Combination of sedation and regional anaesthesia

There is increasing use of regional anaesthesia, but hypovolaemia must be corrected preoperatively. Sedation should not be confused with general anaesthesia. The sedated patient can talk to the anaesthetist at all times. If not, then airway control may be lost, with the risk of aspiration of gastric contents.

23.1 Full stomach

Patients for elective surgery are usually starved for 6 hours to ensure an empty stomach, but can receive clear fluids for up to 2 hours before induction of anaesthesia. Nevertheless, every few years we have the unpleasant experience of dealing with elective patients who vomit undigested food at least 12 hours after the meal in the absence of any intestinal abnormalities. In emergency surgery the 6-hour rule is unreliable, and all emergency patients should be treated as having a full stomach and so at risk of vomiting, regurgitation and aspiration.

Vomiting occurs at the induction of, and emergence from, anaesthesia. If gastric acid enters the lungs a pneumonitis results, which can be fatal. Aspiration can also occur following passive regurgitation of gastric contents up the oesophagus. This regurgitation is often described as 'silent' to distinguish it from active vomiting. Regurgitation is particularly likely at induction of anaesthesia, when several drugs used (atropine, thiopentone, suxamethonium) decrease the pressure in the lower oesophageal sphincter.

In emergency anaesthesia there is always a risk of aspiration, regardless of the period of starvation. Therefore, the trachea must be intubated as rapidly as possible after induction of anaesthesia. The methods available are shown in Box 23.3. If preoperative assessment of the airway indicates no problems then tracheal intubation is performed under general anaesthesia. However, *if a difficult airway is predicted then senior help must be called.*

Box 23.3 Methods of facilitating tracheal intubation

- Patient awake
  - topical anaesthesia with fibreoptic intubation
- Patient anaesthetised
  - use of muscle relaxants
    - suxamethonium
    - non-depolarising relaxants
  - inhalational techniques

There are some basic requirements for tracheal intubation in emergency surgery:
- skilled assistance must be present
- the trolley must tip
- the suction apparatus must work correctly and be left on
- a range of sizes of tracheal tubes must be available
- spare laryngoscopes must be available
- ancillary intubation aids, bougies and stillettes must be available

A plan of management of the patient who may have a full stomach and is at risk of aspiration is shown in Box 23.4.

Box 23.4 Management of tracheal intubation when risk of aspiration

- Empty stomach
  - from above by nasogastric tube
  - from below by drugs, e.g. metoclopramide
- Neutralise remaining stomach contents
  - antacids
  - H_2 blocking drugs to prevent further acid secretion
- Stop central nervous system induced vomiting
  - avoid opioids
  - use phenothiazines
- CORRECT ANAESTHETIC TECHNIQUE
  - 'rapid sequence induction'
  - preoxygenation, cricoid pressure, intubation

Neither physical nor pharmacological methods should be relied on to empty the stomach completely. In some specialties such as obstetrics, an H_2 receptor blocking drug, ranitidine, is given routinely to decrease gastric acid secretion and 30 ml sodium citrate is used orally 15 minutes before induction of anaesthesia to increase the pH of the gastric contents. Opioids delay gastric emptying and increase the likelihood of vomiting.

The only reliable way to prevent regurgitation is to use the correct anaesthetic technique. This is now called a rapid sequence induction, which sounds better than the old term – crash induction. It has three essential components: preoxygenation, cricoid pressure, intubation.

Preoxygenation

Before induction the patient must breathe 100% oxygen for at least 3 minutes from a suitable breathing circuit. There should be no leaks and the flow rate of oxygen in the circuit should be high to prevent rebreathing. Air contains oxygen, nitrogen and minimal carbon dioxide. When the patient is breathing oxygen only, the lungs denitrogenate rapidly and after 3 minutes contain only oxygen and carbon dioxide. There is now a greater reservoir of oxygen in the lungs to utilise before hypoxia occurs.

Anaesthesia is then induced and cricoid pressure applied.

Cricoid pressure

The cricoid cartilage is identified on the patient before anaesthesia is induced and the patient is warned that they might feel pressure on the neck as they go to sleep. The skilled assistant presses down on the cricoid cartilage as anaesthesia is induced and *this pressure is applied continuously until the anaesthetist tells the assistant to stop* (Figure 23.1).

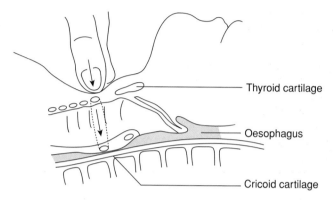

Figure 23.1 Application of cricoid pressure.

The object of pressure on the cricoid cartilage is to compress the oesophagus between the cricoid cartilage and vertebral column. This prevents any material that has been regurgitated from the stomach into the oesophagus from passing into the pharynx.

Cricoid pressure is usually undertaken by firm, but gentle, pressure on the cartilage by the thumb and forefinger of the assistant. It is similar to the pressure exerted that causes mild pain when the thumb and forefinger are pressed onto the bridge of the nose. The cricoid cartilage is used because it is easily identifiable, forms a complete tracheal ring, and the trachea is not distorted when it is compressed.

The patient has now received preoxygenation, an induction agent, and cricoid pressure. A neuromuscular blocking drug is given to facilitate intubation of the trachea.

Intubation

The neuromuscular blocking drug must act rapidly and have a short duration of action. The lungs are not ventilated during a rapid sequence induction; this will prevent accidental inflation of the stomach, which will further predispose the patient to regurgitation and vomiting. Gases can be forced into the oesophagus and stomach during manual ventilation of the lungs despite the application of cricoid pressure.

A drug with a rapid onset of action permits quick tracheal intubation. An agent with a short duration of action is valuable because in cases of failed intubation spontaneous respiration will return promptly. This allows other options to be considered (Chapter 4).

Suxamethonium has many side effects (Box 23.5) but remains the best drug available.

Box 23.5 Major side effects of suxamethonium

- Muscle pain
- Bradycardia
- Raised intracranial pressure
- Raised intraocular pressure
- Raised intragastric pressure
- Allergic reactions
- Hyperkalaemia in burns, paraplegia, some myopathies
- Prolonged action in pseudocholinesterase deficiency
- Malignant hyperthermia

Only when the trachea is intubated, the cuff inflated and the correct position of the tube confirmed, is the cricoid pressure released.

The anaesthetic is maintained, usually with a volatile agent, oxygen, non-depolarising relaxant and suitable analgesia. The reversal of the relaxant at the end of the procedure is undertaken with the anticholinesterase, neostigmine. Glycopyrrolate is given concomitantly to stop bradycardia occurring from the neostigmine.

Rapid sequence induction has the major disadvantage of potential haemodynamic instability, as hypertension and tachycardia often occur following laryngoscopy and intubation. This is often more severe than in elective surgery when opioids are given at induction of anaesthesia.

23.2 Other indications for rapid sequence induction

Every anaesthetic, not just emergency work, should be considered from the point of view of unexpected vomiting or regurgitation. Some cases are at high risk, and rapid sequence induction should be considered carefully as an option in this group (Box 23.6).

Box 23.6 High risk factors for regurgitation

- Oesophageal disease
  - pouch
  - stricture
- Gastro-oesophageal sphincter abnormalities
  - hiatus hernia
  - obesity
  - drugs
- Gastric emptying delay
  - trauma
  - pyloric stenosis
  - gastric malignancy
  - opioids
  - patient predisposition, anxiety
  - pregnancy
  - recent food intake
- Abnormal bowel peristalsis
  - peritonitis
  - ileus – metabolic or drugs
  - bowel obstruction

23.3 Pulmonary aspiration

Pulmonary aspiration may be obvious. The presence of lager and curry in the pharynx when the blade of the laryngoscope is inserted is a depressing sight. It may also be silent, presenting as a postoperative pulmonary complication.

The signs of pulmonary aspiration are shown in Box 23.7.

Box 23.7 Signs of pulmonary aspiration

- None
- Oxygen desaturation
- Coughing
- Tachypnoea
- Unexplained tachycardia
- Wheeze
- Hypotension
- Pneumonitis
- Postoperative pulmonary disease

Treatment requires the advice of a senior anaesthetist. The airway must be suctioned and *oxygenation of the patient remains the priority*. Bronchoscopy may be required to remove particulate matter. If the patient is not paralysed then, surgery permitting, he or she should be allowed to wake up. If paralysed, intubation and ventilation must occur and oxygenation maintained.

Bronchospasm may be treated with salbutanol or aminophylline. Further treatment may include antibiotics, other bronchodilators and steroids. Aggressive early management is required.

23.4 Postoperative care

Always plan the postoperative care of the patient. Inform the ward, high dependency unit or intensive care unit of your needs for the patient (Box 23.8).

Box 23.8 Levels of care

- Level 0   Patients whose needs can be met through normal ward care in an acute hospital
- Level 1   Patients at risk of their condition deteriorating, or those recently relocated from higher levels of care whose needs can be met on an acute ward with additional advice and support from the critical care team
- Level 2   Patients requiring more detailed observation or intervention including support for a single failing organ or postoperative care, and those stepping down from high levels of care
- Level 3   Patients requiring advanced respiratory support alone or basic respiratory support together with support of at least two organs. This level includes all complex patients requiring support for multi-organ failure

HDU can be level 1 or 2
ICU can be level 2 or 3

23.5 Conclusion

Anaesthesia for emergency surgery needs careful preoperative assessment, and adequate resuscitation must be undertaken before surgery.

Impatient surgeons must be restrained. A rapid sequence induction of anaesthesia must follow the order of preoxygenation, cricoid pressure and intubation to prevent aspiration of gastric contents.

Chapter 24 **Epidural and spinal anaesthesia**

Before undertaking regional anaesthesia, the criteria outlined in Box 24.1 must be considered and satisfied.

Box 24.1 Requirements before starting regional anaesthesia

- Informed consent
- Vascular access
- Resuscitation drugs and equipment
- Sterility of anaesthetist
- Sterility of operative site
- No contraindications to procedure
- Correct dosage of local anaesthetic drug

Sterility of the anaesthetist does not refer to his or her reproductive capacity, but means wearing a gown, mask, hat and gloves.

24.1 Epidural anaesthesia

The epidural space runs from the base of the skull to the bottom of the sacrum at the sacrococcygeal membrane. The spinal cord, cerebrospinal fluid and meninges are enclosed within it (Figure 24.1).

The spinal cord becomes the cauda equina at the level of L2 in an adult and the cerebrospinal fluid stops at the level of S2. The epidural space is 3–6 mm wide and is defined posteriorly by the ligamentum flavum, the anterior surfaces of the vertebral laminae, and the articular processes. Anteriorly it is related to the posterior longitudinal ligament and laterally is bounded by the intervertebral foramina and the pedicles.

How to Survive in Anaesthesia: A Guide for Trainees, Fourth Edition.
Neville Robinson, George Hall and William Fawcett.
© 2012 John Wiley & Sons, Ltd. Published 2012 by John Wiley & Sons, Ltd.

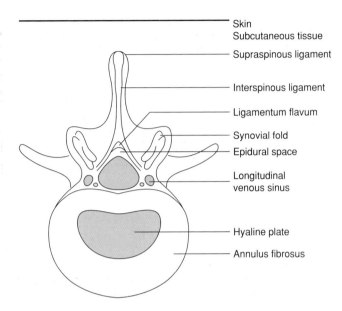

Skin
Subcutaneous tissue
Supraspinous ligament

Interspinous ligament

Ligamentum flavum

Synovial fold
Epidural space

Longitudinal
venous sinus

Hyaline plate

Annulus fibrosus

Figure 24.1 Anatomy of the epidural space.

The contents of the epidural space are:
- nerve roots
- venous plexus
- fat
- lymphatics

The veins contain no valves and communicate directly with the intracranial, thoracic and abdominal venous systems.

Contraindications to epidural anaesthesia are shown in Box 24.2. Abnormal clotting may result in haemorrhage in a confined space if an epidural vein is punctured during the insertion of an epidural cannula. An epidural haematoma then causes spinal cord compression. Local skin infection may introduce bacteria into the spinal meninges with the risk of an abscess or meningitis. Similarly with septicaemia – if a vein is punctured then the small haematoma is a good culture medium for bacteria.

Box 24.2 Absolute and relative contraindications to epidural anaesthesia

- Absolute
  - patient refusal
  - abnormal clotting

- infection – local on back, septicaemia
- allergy to local anaesthetic drug
• Relative
  - raised intracranial pressure
  - hypovolaemia
  - chronic spinal disorders
  - central nervous system disease
  - drugs – aspirin, other NSAIDs, low-dose heparin
  - fixed cardiac output states e.g. aortic stenosis

Although the evidence that spinal disorders are exacerbated by the insertion of an epidural catheter is poor, patients are often quick to blame the anaesthetic procedure. The same principle applies to patients with neurological problems such as multiple sclerosis. The evidence that drugs that mildly affect clotting or platelet function (for example, non-steroidal anti-inflammatory drugs) cause abnormal bleeding in the epidural space and increase the risk of an epidural haematoma is minimal.

The equipment used for the insertion of an epidural catheter is shown in Figure 24.2.

The Tuohy needle is either 16 or 18 gauge. It is 10 cm long: 8 cm of needle and 2 cm of hub. It is marked in centimetres and has a curved 'Huber' tip. The epidural catheter has three holes at 120° alignment, with the holes 2 cm from the end of the catheter. The catheter is marked in centimetre gradations up to 20 cm. The filter has a 0.2 μm mesh that stops the injection of particulate matter, such as glass, and bacteria into the epidural space.

The correct technique of insertion of an epidural catheter must be learnt under careful supervision. The conditions listed in Box 24.2 must be met. An intravenous infusion of either crystalloid or colloid is set up to give a 'fluid load' of about 500 ml before the local anaesthetic is injected. This is undertaken to decrease the likelihood of hypotension with the onset of the epidural block. Atropine and a vasopressor should always be drawn up before starting the block.

The procedure can be done in either the lateral or sitting position, and ideally the spine should be flexed. A slow, controlled advance of the Tuohy needle is essential, using a syringe and a loss-of-resistance technique. The needle passes through skin, subcutaneous tissue, supraspinous ligament, interspinous ligament, ligamentum flavum, and finally enters the epidural space. The ligaments resist the injection of air or saline, but when the needle enters the epidural space the resistance is lost.

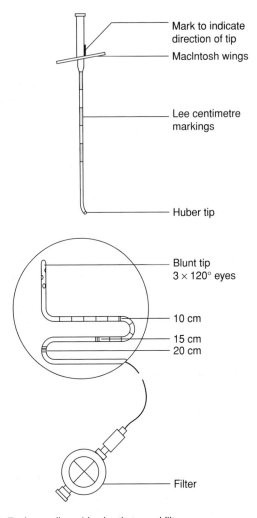

Figure 24.2 Tuohy needle, epidural catheter and filter.

The choice is between using air or saline to identify the epidural space. The *advantages of air* are that:
- any fluid in the needle or catheter must be cerebrospinal fluid
- there is less equipment on the tray
- it is cheaper

The *disadvantages of air* are that:
- injection of large volumes may result in patchy blockade
- there is a theoretical risk of air embolus

The *advantages of saline* are that:
• it is a more reliable method of identifying the epidural space
• the catheter passes more easily into epidural space
The *disadvantages of saline* are that:
• fluid in the needle or catheter may be either saline or cerebrospinal fluid; the latter is warmer and contains glucose, but rapid clinical decisions are difficult
• there are additional fluids on the tray, with increased risk of error
We recommend you become thoroughly familiar with either air or saline before trying the alternative method. There is no 'correct' method; one author uses air and the others use saline.

The epidural space is usually found at a distance of about 4–6 cm from the skin. Place the catheter rostrally and, using the centimetre markings on the needle and catheter, insert 3 cm of catheter into the epidural space.

The filter and catheter, once correctly positioned and fixed, must be aspirated to ensure that no blood or cerebrospinal fluid can be withdrawn. The local anaesthetic drug is given in small, incremental doses to reduce the risk of complications.

The complications of epidural blockade, assuming no technical difficulties in the location of the space and the siting of the catheter, are shown in Boxes 24.3 and 24.4.

Box 24.3 Major complications of epidural anaesthesia

• Severe hypotension
• Accidental intravenous injection
• Dural puncture
  − massive spinal anaesthetic
  − headache

Box 24.4 Other complications of epidural anaesthesia

• Leg weakness
• Shivering
• Atonic bladder
• Contraction of the small bowel
• Backache
• Isolated, reversible nerve damage from catheter/needle trauma
• Epidural haematoma
• Epidural abscess
• Meningitis

Hypotension results from a decreased venous return to the heart as a consequence of vasodilation induced by the sympathetic blockade. The 'fluid load' helps to prevent hypotension, but a vasoconstrictor, such as ephedrine in 3–6 mg intravenous increments, is often given to restore normal arterial pressure.

The risks of the intravenous injection of local anaesthetic are minimised by aspiration of the catheter and by giving small incremental doses. If blood is aspirated, usually the catheter is removed and the epidural resited in a different space. Occasionally, the catheter can be withdrawn from the epidural vein and no blood aspirated. Then the catheter must be flushed with saline to ensure it is not in a vein before further use.

Accidental dural puncture occurs when the needle or catheter is inserted into the cerebrospinal fluid. If this is not recognised and a full epidural dose of local anaesthetic is injected into the wrong place, a massive spinal anaesthetic will result, with apnoea, severe hypotension and total paralysis. The lungs have to be ventilated and the circulation supported during this period. For this reason, an epidural 'test dose' of 2–3 ml of local anaesthetic is given by many anaesthetists before the full dose is injected (for example, 2% lignocaine). In the epidural space this dose of local anaesthetic has little effect, but in the cerebrospinal fluid an extensive block occurs rapidly. After 10 minutes the epidural dose of local anaesthetic is given if no adverse effects are noted.

A severe postural headache following dural puncture is managed by resting the patient in a flat position, simple analgesics, adequate hydration, caffeine and, if necessary, a 'blood patch'. The dural puncture can be sealed by placing 20 ml of the patient's blood into the epidural space under aseptic conditions. The resulting clot will rapidly stop the leak and is effective in virtually all patients. Two anaesthetists are required for this manoeuvre.

Opioids can also be given in the epidural space to prolong the effects of local anaesthetics and to provide postoperative analgesia. They have different complications (Box 24.5), of which respiratory depression is the most serious. Regular monitoring of respiratory function is essential (see Chapter 31).

Box 24.5 Complications of epidural opioids

- Delayed respiratory depression
- Drowsiness
- Itchiness
- Nausea and vomiting
- Urinary retention

24.2 Spinal anaesthesia

This is the deliberate injection of local anaesthetic into the cerebrospinal fluid (CSF) by means of a lumbar puncture. It is normally given as a single injection, but can be used in conjunction with epidural anaesthesia (combined spinal–epidural anaesthesia) for longer procedures.

The incidence of headache following dural puncture is dependent on the size and type of spinal needle. Not surprisingly, the smaller the diameter of the needle, the lower the incidence of headache (remember, 27 gauge is *smaller* than 25 gauge).

Pencil-tip spinal needles, such as Whitacre and Sprotte, split, rather than cut, the dura and also reduce the risk of headache.

Local anaesthetic solutions for spinal anaesthesia are isobaric or hyperbaric with respect to the CSF. Isobaric solutions are claimed to have a more predictable spread in the CSF, independent of the position of the patient. Hyperbaric solutions are produced by the addition of glucose, and their spread is partially influenced by gravity. Many factors determine the distribution of local anaesthetic solutions in the CSF (Box 24.6); this makes prediction of the level of blockade difficult.

Box 24.6 Factors influencing distribution of local anaesthetic solutions in CSF

- Patient age
- Local anaesthetic drug
- Baricity
- Dose of drug
- Volume of drug
- Turbulence of cerebrospinal fluid
- Increased abdominal pressure
- Spinal curvatures
- Position of patient
- Use of vasoconstrictors
- Speed of injection

The complications of spinal anaesthesia are the same as for epidural anaesthesia. Neuronal blockade is more rapid in onset, so the side effects, such as hypotension, occur promptly. In spinal anaesthesia the duration of the block is variable, but it is usually shorter than that of epidural anaesthesia.

24.3 Caudal anaesthesia

The caudal space is a continuation of the epidural space in the sacral region. The signet-shaped sacral hiatus is formed by the failure of fusion of the laminae of the fifth sacral vertebra. The hiatus is bounded laterally by the sacral cornua and is covered by the posterior sacrococcygeal ligament, subcutaneous tissue and skin. The epidural space is located by passing a needle through the sacral hiatus. The caudal canal contains veins, fat and the sacral nerves. The cerebrospinal fluid finishes at the level of S2.

Caudal anaesthesia is used for operations in areas supplied by the sacral nerves, such as anal surgery and circumcision. The precautions are the same as those described for epidural anaesthesia. The needle must be aspirated after insertion to exclude blood and cerebrospinal fluid. The complications are the same as for epidural anaesthesia, although motor blockade can be a major problem in the early postoperative period if the patient wants to walk.

Hypotension is uncommon, as the neuronal blockade usually does not spread rostrally to reach the sympathetic chain.

The extent of a block can be measured by the absence of pain or temperature sensation at a dermatomal level (Table 24.1). The former is tested with a sharp needle and the latter with an ethyl chloride spray.

Table 24.1 Dermatomal levels at various anatomical landmarks

Anatomical landmark	Dermatomal level
Nipples	T4
Xiphisternum	T6
Umbilicus	T10
Symphysis pubis	L1/T12

24.4 Conclusion

Regional anaesthesia is fun for the anaesthetist and provides excellent analgesia for the patient. The successful use of these techniques depends on learning good technical skills to match understanding of essential anatomy, physiology and pharmacology.

Start early in your career – make the epidural space a familiar territory.

Chapter 25 **Anaesthesia for gynaecological surgery**

Gynaecological surgery is undertaken for diagnostic and therapeutic reasons. The trainee anaesthetist is often introduced to anaesthesia by means of supervised teaching on routine gynaecology lists. Laparoscopic procedures are common in gynaecological surgery, general surgery and urology.

25.1 Laparoscopy

Laparoscopy requires the formation of a pneumoperitoneum, and carbon dioxide is used as the insufflating gas for reasons shown in Box 25.1.

Box 25.1 Advantages of CO_2 use for pneumoperitoneum

- Cheap
- Readily available
- Non-toxic
- Does not support combustion
- More soluble in blood than air (20 ×)
- Buffered by formation of bicarbonate
- Easily excreted by the lungs

There are three main anaesthetic considerations when surgery is conducted laparoscopically:
- problems from gas insufflation
- trauma by Veress needle or trochar
- anaesthetic complications

How to Survive in Anaesthesia: A Guide for Trainees, Fourth Edition.
Neville Robinson, George Hall and William Fawcett.
© 2012 John Wiley & Sons, Ltd. Published 2012 by John Wiley & Sons, Ltd.

Problems from gas insufflation

When carbon dioxide is insufflated to cause the pneumoperitoneum, physiological changes occur (Box 25.2).

Box 25.2 Problems arising from gas insufflation

• Cardiovascular changes
• Respiratory changes
• Cardiac arrhythmias
• Misplacement of the insufflating gas
• Gas embolism
• Hypothermia

Insufflation pressures of 10–15 mm Hg are well tolerated, but pressures greater than 30 mm Hg can result in profound haemodynamic responses. The pneumoperitoneum increases intra-abdominal and intrathoracic pressures. This decreases venous return and so lowers cardiac output. In contrast, carbon dioxide absorption increases sympathetic activity to augment cardiac contractility and increase heart rate. During anaesthesia there is usually a satisfactory circulation with a normal or raised arterial blood pressure and a tachycardia. Problems arise, however, when haemorrhage occurs, as the usual compensatory cardiovascular responses may be inadequate.

Diaphragmatic splinting can result in basal atelectasis, increased intrapulmonary shunts, hypoxia and hypercarbia in spontaneously breathing patients. These changes are minimised by positive pressure ventilation.

Cardiac arrhythmias may result from a low cardiac output in the presence of hypercarbia.

Inadvertent misplacement of the insufflating gas can cause subcutaneous emphysema, pneumomediastinum, pneumothorax and pneumopericardium. Although rare, we have seen all these complications, with the exception of a pneumopericardium.

Carbon dioxide gas embolism is a major complication, as a large embolus will cause outflow obstruction of the pulmonary artery. The diagnosis is made by the occurrence of sudden hypotension, hypoxia and a low expired carbon dioxide tension.

Hypothermia may occur in long procedures. A 0.3 °C decrease in core temperature has been found for each 50 litres of carbon dioxide insufflated.

Trauma by Veress needle or trochar

Major damage can occur (Box 25.3).

Box 25.3 Complications from needle or trochar insertion

- Haemorrhage
- Intestinal perforation
- Other visceral trauma

Haemorrhage can result from the passage of the trochar or needle through the anterior abdominal wall. Tearing of adhesions from the expanding pneumoperitoneum will also cause bleeding. Traumatic puncture of the major intra-abdominal vessels has been reported. One author observed a large tear in the internal iliac artery, which was ultimately fatal. The raised intra-abdominal pressure may tamponade even a large vessel, and venous haemorrhage may not be obvious during the laparoscopy, leading to a delay in a subsequent laparotomy.

Intestinal perforation can occur. The bowel can be grazed, leading to peritonitis, abscess formation and sepsis. Puncture of the bladder, ureters and liver has been reported.

In summary, if an organ is in the peritoneal cavity, then it has been damaged at laparoscopy.

Anaesthetic problems associated with laparoscopy

There are several implications for the anaesthetist of laparoscopic surgery. These are listed in Box 25.4.

Box 25.4 Anaesthetic problems of laparoscopic surgery

- Aspiration of gastric contents
- Position of patient
- Nerve injury
- Conversion to laparotomy
- Postoperative pain relief
- Anaesthetic technique

It is often assumed that the Trendelenberg position and a pneumoperitoneum will lead to an increased risk of passive regurgitation of gastric contents. However, the lower oesophageal sphincter pressure alters little and the risk, although present, is low.

The patient is often in a steep Trendelenberg position for gynaecological surgery, but may be in a head-up position for abdominal surgery. Occasionally, both are employed in the same patient.

Nerve damage can occur: the common peroneal nerve, femoral nerve and the brachial plexus are at risk.

A small number of patients proceed to laparotomy. The anaesthetist should be prepared for this possibility at the start of the procedure.

Postoperative pain can be decreased by infiltrating the wounds made by the trochar with local anaesthetic. Shoulder tip pain may occur from diaphragmatic irritation by the gas.

Many anaesthetic techniques have been used for laparoscopy. Epidural and spinal anaesthesia are not well tolerated because of the discomfort from peritoneal distension and respiratory stimulation. General anaesthesia is used frequently. The safest and preferred technique is tracheal intubation and ventilation of the patient. This allows abdominal wall relaxation and decreases the effects of diaphragmatic splinting on respiratory function. The risk of gastric aspiration is minimised – and, should a laparotomy ensue, you are prepared. Emergency laparoscopic surgery necessitates a rapid sequence induction technique. Adequate venous access is essential for laparoscopic surgery, as brisk haemorrhage can occur.

25.2 Ectopic pregnancy

Ectopic pregnancy is sometimes a life-threatening emergency. The relevant anaesthetic considerations are shown in Box 25.5.

Box 25.5 Anaesthetic considerations in ectopic pregnancy

- Patient empathy
- Emergency anaesthesia
- Haemorrhage
- Pregnancy
- Surgical technique – laparotomy or laparoscopy
- Postoperative analgesia

Patients are often very upset; be kind. There may be considerable blood loss, and full resuscitation should occur before induction of anaesthesia. Adequate blood must be available, but occasionally it is necessary to start surgery without this facility to save life. Insert a wide-bore intravenous cannula before induction; do not rely on a cannula placed by a gynaecologist.

A rapid sequence induction technique is used to avoid gastric aspiration. The surgical procedure may be done by a laparotomy, or by a laparoscopic technique. Appropriate postoperative analgesia should be prescribed.

Case study
A 32-year-old woman is pale, sweaty, with lower abdominal pain. Her heart rate is 120/minute and BP 75/40. The diagnosis is ruptured ectopic pregancy for emergency laparatomy.

Preoperative care
Oxygen, large-bore IV access, cross-match 4 units of blood, give rapid, warmed IV fluid until blood is available. May require CVP and urinary catheter.

Perioperative care
Induction. Rapid sequence. Cardiovascular stable agents. Arterial cannula may be required.
Maintenance. Ensure BP, heart rate and temperature are maintained in normal range.

Postoperative care
Will require close monitoring, including CVP and urine output, to check for fluid status. If massive blood transfusion, will require check haemoglobin and clotting screen postoperatively. Check chest x-ray for CVP, if used. Check ABGs for acidosis and lactate. Pain control, e.g. PCA. Will require oxygen for 12 hours.

25.3 Evacuation of retained products of conception (ERPC)

This operation is very common, and the anaesthetic considerations are shown in Box 25.6.

Box 25.6 Anaesthetic considerations for ERPC

- Patient empathy
- Timing of surgery
- Pregnancy
- Haemorrhage
- Oxytocic drugs
- Infection

> • Type of anaesthesia
>   – regional or general
>   – need for tracheal intubation

Again a sympathetic approach to the patient is essential. An ERPC is not an emergency procedure and, in the absence of haemorrhage, should be undertaken during routine operating time. The risks of the procedure are haemorrhage, infection and uterine perforation. Oxytocic drugs are used to contract the uterus. Syntocinon is commonly used as a bolus injection and occasionally causes hypotension. Ergometrine contracts smooth muscle and can provoke vomiting.

Regional anaesthesia can be used for ERPC (epidural, spinal) and a level of analgesia to T10 is required. Usually the surgery is carried out under general anaesthesia. There are two special considerations. The first relates to the pregnant patient and the full stomach. If the procedure is not an emergency, the patient is not suffering from any specific symptoms of pregnancy, such as heartburn, and the patient is less than 16 weeks pregnant, then tracheal intubation is unnecessary. If the patient is more than 16 weeks pregnant, a rapid sequence induction and tracheal intubation is recommended.

Moreover, volatile anaesthetic agents relax the uterus. This increases blood loss and the risk of perforation of the uterus. Therefore, some anaesthetists will not use volatile agents. Instead, intravenous anaesthesia (propofol) with supplementation by nitrous oxide and oxygen is given.

25.4 Laparotomy

General anaesthesia for operations on the uterus and the ovaries is similar to that described in abdominal anaesthesia (Chapter 27).

Regional anaesthesia is an excellent technique for gynaecological surgery, with the benefit of good postoperative analgesia. The innervation of the uterus is up to T10. If manipulation of the bowel occurs, or if there is haemorrhage in the paracolic gutters, the patient may experience discomfort. An extension of neural blockade to T4 (as for a Caesarean section) is then needed to relieve pain.

25.5 Hysteroscopy

In this procedure clear irrigating fluid is used to expand the uterus and allow telescopic visualisation of the contents. Although the risks are usually slight, acute water intoxication can occur (see Chapter 26, Box 26.4).

25.6 Conclusion

You will undertake a lot of anaesthesia for gynaecological surgery in the early months of your career. Always assume that the gynaecologists have no knowledge of anything that occurs outside the pelvis, preoperative assessment must be meticulous, and do not underestimate their ability to cause severe blood loss.

Chapter 26 **Anaesthesia for urological surgery**

Urological surgical lists provide supervised experience in anaesthetising elderly patients with medical problems. They are useful for learning basic regional techniques such as spinal anaesthesia.

26.1 Transurethral resection of the prostate (TURP)

This involves resection of the prostate by a modified cystoscope, which cuts tissue and coagulates blood vessels. The procedure is facilitated by means of irrigating fluid that flows through the cystoscope. This fluid washes blood away from the cut prostatic tissue so that the operative site can be seen. Further resection occurs and any bleeding venous sinuses are coagulated. The requirements of the irrigating fluid are shown in Box 26.1.

Box 26.1 Requirements for urological irrigating fluid

- Prevents dispersal of electrical current
- Clear for visibility
- Sterile
- Non-toxic locally
- Non-toxic systemically
- Isothermic
- Isotonic
- Non-haemolytic
- Inexpensive

The current from the diathermy must not be spread to the bladder wall through the irrigating fluid. The fluid must be non-toxic, especially if

---

How to Survive in Anaesthesia: A Guide for Trainees, Fourth Edition.
Neville Robinson, George Hall and William Fawcett.
© 2012 John Wiley & Sons, Ltd. Published 2012 by John Wiley & Sons, Ltd.

absorbed through the open venous sinuses of the prostate. The solution used in current practice is glycine 1.5%, which is slightly hypotonic (2.1% is isotonic).

Irrigation is performed under hydrostatic pressure during prostatic resection, and some intravenous absorption of the glycine will take place through the prostatic venous sinuses. The amount of irrigating fluid absorbed depends on several factors (Box 26.2).

Box 26.2 Factors influencing the absorption of glycine

- Hydrostatic pressure of the irrigating fluid
- Number and size of the venous sinuses opened
- Duration of surgery
- Venous pressure at the irrigant–blood interface

The height of the glycine should be less than 70 cm above the patient. Symptoms of glycine absorption may take as little as 15 minutes to appear, and up to 2 litres of fluid can be absorbed. Usually surgery is restricted to a duration of 1 hour only.

Anaesthetic considerations for TURP are shown in Box 26.3.

Box 26.3 Anaesthetic problems for TURP

- Elderly population
- Concurrent diseases
- Dilutional hyponatraemia and overhydration (TURP syndrome)
- Haemolysis
- Haemorrhage
- Infection
- Patient position
- Hypothermia
- Perforation of bladder
- Erection
- Adductor spasm
- Burns and explosions
- Postoperative clot retention

Elderly men often have severe medical problems, which must be assessed and treated preoperatively. If prostatic obstruction is chronic, renal impairment may be present.

TURP syndrome

The absorption intravenously of the irrigating fluid, if severe, causes iatrogenic water intoxication – the TURP syndrome. This can present in a number of ways and is more easily detected in an awake patient having regional anaesthesia than in one undergoing general anaesthesia. Symptoms and signs of the TURP syndrome are shown in Box 26.4.

Box 26.4 Symptoms and signs of acute water intoxication (TURP syndrome)

- Agitation
- Restlessness
- Confusion
- Vomiting
- Blurred vision
- Transient blindness
- Coma
- Convulsions
- Unexplained bradycardia
- Unexplained hypotension
- Unexplained hypertension
- Pulmonary oedema
- ECG changes
- Asystole

Signs of cerebral irritation are usually seen first, and vomiting is a consistent feature. Under general anaesthesia ECG changes, such as a wide QRS complex, T-wave inversion, and rarely ventricular tachycardia and asystole, may be the only signs.

If water intoxication is suspected, the blood tests shown in Box 26.5 should be done immediately.

Box 26.5 Blood tests in suspected TURP syndrome

- Haemoglobin/haematocrit
- Serum osmolality
- Plasma sodium
- Plasma potassium
- Plasma glycine
- Plasma ammonia

The most important findings are a low plasma sodium concentration, low osmolality and low haemoglobin concentration. A sodium concentration of less than 120 mmol/l is associated with significant symptoms and signs. The plasma ammonia and glycine values will not be immediately available, but will confirm the absorption of the glycine.

Treatment should be aimed at prevention and then management of the syndrome (Box 26.6). Treatment of acute intoxication is undertaken rapidly; the prompt reversal of *chronic* water intoxication can result in cerebral pontine myelosis.

Box 26.6 Management of water intoxication in TURP syndrome

- Prevention
  - correct intravenous fluid of choice (avoid 5% glucose, glucose/saline solutions)
  - short duration of surgery by competent surgeon
- Treatment
  - stop surgery if possible
  - oxygen
  - CVP measurement
  - diuresis
  - intravenous sodium solutions
  - circulatory support
  - symptom control
  - may require ventilation

Sodium chloride solution (0.9%) or colloids are the intravenous fluid of choice for TURP.

The TURP syndrome is a medical emergency and needs experienced anaesthetic help. Diuretic therapy is the mainstay of treatment and frusemide is the agent of choice; 0.9% sodium chloride or even hypertonic saline should be given judiciously to increase the plasma sodium concentration.

Other anaesthetic problems

Haemolysis presents in a similar way to a transfusion reaction. The patient may complain of weakness, rigors and chest pain, and become hypertensive. Haemoglobinaemia, haemoglobinuria and anaemia may occur, with acute tubular necrosis. Treatment should be directed towards obtaining a diuresis and specific correction of the haematological and biochemical abnormalities.

Haemorrhage is not uncommon, and blood loss is difficult to assess since the blood is diluted with irrigating fluid. The usual methods of estimating blood loss are inappropriate. Careful assessment of the circulation by conventional means is used. If methods of estimating the haemoglobin concentration of the irrigating fluid are available, then the blood loss can be calculated.

Bacteraemia and septicaemia can result from instrumentation, and there is always the risk of sudden postoperative septicaemia. Antibiotics, especially gentamicin, are given on induction to reduce this risk.

The patient is in the lithotomy position, which assists venous return. When the patient's legs are placed horizontally at the end of surgery, especially when regional techniques are used, the arterial pressure often declines as a result of the decreased venous return.

Irrigating fluids during prolonged surgery cause hypothermia. Occasionally, perforation of the bladder can occur.

Erection, which usually occurs when regional anaesthesia is used, prevents instrumentation of the penis and surgery is not possible. Ketamine in small incremental doses of 5–10 mg intravenously is reputed to help with this irritating and embarrassing problem.

If the obturator nerve is stimulated accidentally by the surgeon, adductor spasm occurs. Sudden closure of the thighs commands the attention of the surgeon.

There is always a slight risk of burns and explosions, since the diathermy carries high-frequency current at a power of up to 400 W with a voltage of 2000 V.

If clot retention occurs postoperatively, the urinary catheter will block. The irrigating fluid must be turned off until the clot is removed by flushing the catheter and bladder. If the irrigating fluid is kept running, the bladder will fill and the irrigating fluid will be absorbed through the prostatic venous plexus. This is painful and dangerous, with the risk of TURP syndrome.

The operation is not usually painful and, after regional anaesthesia, little further pain relief is needed.

The choices of anaesthesia for TURP are shown in Box 26.7.

Box 26.7 Anaesthesia for TURP

• Regional anaesthesia (± sedation)
  − spinal
  − epidural
• General anaesthesia
  − spontaneous ventilation
  − controlled ventilation

Regional anaesthesia must reach the level of T10 to prevent pain from bladder distension. General and regional anaesthesia are sometimes combined.

The advantages and disadvantages of regional anaesthesia are shown in Box 26.8.

Box 26.8 Advantages and disadvantages of regional anaesthesia for TURP

- Advantages
  - avoids complications of general anaesthesia
  - better postoperative analgesia
  - early recognition of TURP syndrome
  - less deep vein thrombosis
  - earlier mobilisation
  - less bleeding intraoperatively
  - better operating field
- Disadvantages
  - less control of arterial pressure
  - headaches
  - difficult to position elderly patient for block
  - patient preference for unconsciousness

The advantages and disadvantages of general anaesthesia are shown in Box 26.9.

Box 26.9 Advantages and disadvantages of general anaesthesia for TURP

- Advantages
  - often faster
  - patient preference
  - surgeon preference
  - better control of arterial pressure
  - avoids complications of regional anaesthesia
- Disadvantages
  - slower recovery period
  - postoperative analgesia less good
  - slower mobilisation
  - slower recognition of TURP syndrome
  - risk of general anaesthetic complications

Case study

A 72-year-old man presents for TURP with a 2-week history of chronic retention with overflow. He also has atrial fibrillation at a rate of 120/minute and takes aspirin, and ramipril for hypertension.

Preoperative care

Patient may have some renal impairment (and hyperkalaemia) from earlier ureteric obstruction with anaemia. The AF rate should be controlled to approx 80–90/minute preoperatively. Consider spinal anaesthesia. Continue aspirin.

Perioperative care

Induction. Choice of regional or general anaesthesia – see Boxes 26.8 and 26.9.

Maintenance. Ensure blood pressure is maintained to prevent further deterioration in renal function. Avoid nephrotoxic drugs (gentamicin/NSAIDs). Fluid replacement (including blood if required) is essential, particularly when the legs are lowered, as hypotension can occur.

Postoperative care

Watch for haemorrhage and TURP syndrome. The latter can complicate prolonged surgery when large amounts of hypotonic solution are absorbed resulting in fluid overload and hyponatraemia, which leads to oedema (cerebral and pulmonary) (Box 26.4). Check urea, electrolytes and haemoglobin postoperatively (Box 26.5).

26.2 Cystoscopic procedures

Cystoscopy can be done with flexible or rigid cystoscopes on an inpatient or outpatient list, under either general or local anaesthesia. Rigid cystoscopy is usually performed under general anaesthesia. The surgical requirement for resection, or biopsy, of the bladder wall is that the patient does not cough or strain unexpectedly, and that respiration is not forced (a smooth anaesthetic with a perfect airway). Otherwise, the bowel will move the bladder wall and there is a risk of perforation. A laparotomy will be required to repair the bladder.

26.3 Circumcision

Circumcision, whether in a child or an adult, is a painful operation, and good postoperative analgesia must be provided. The most common methods are either a caudal anaesthetic, which may result in leg weakness for several hours, or a penile nerve block. For the latter, local anaesthetic is injected in the midline below the symphysis pubis, with the risk of intravascular injection.

26.4 Operations on testicles

Torsion of the testes is a surgical emergency, and appropriate precautions must be undertaken (see Chapter 23). The operation is usually conducted under general anaesthesia. If regional anaesthesia is used, neuronal blockade to the level of T9 is required.

26.5 Renal surgery

Specific problems of renal surgery are shown in Box 26.10.

Box 26.10 Specific considerations in renal surgery

• Position of patient
• Difficult access to intravenous cannulae
• Muscle relaxation
• Haemorrhage
• Pneumothorax
• Postoperative analgesia

The patient may be supine or in a lateral, jack-knife position. Good muscular relaxation is a surgical requirement. Intraoperative haemorrhage may be considerable. The risk of a pneumothorax should not be underestimated (see Chapter 17). Good postoperative analgesia is essential, and epidural analgesia is often used. A combination of general anaesthesia and regional anaesthesia (epidural) is particularly appropriate for renal surgery.

26.6 Conclusion

Urological surgical lists are often unpopular with trainees, but anaesthesia for these patients is challenging. Patients are usually male, elderly, with medical problems, and the surgery has some specific complications.

Careful preoperative assessment is essential and regional anaesthesia is often appropriate. One author spent many happy years helping relieve obstruction in old men.

Chapter 27 **Anaesthesia for abdominal surgery**

27.1 General considerations

Laparoscopic techniques are increasingly common in abdominal surgery, for example laparoscopic cholecystectomy and laparoscopically assisted colectomy. The anaesthetic implications of laparoscopic surgery are discussed in Chapter 25. Careful anaesthetic management of the patient is essential in abdominal surgery, as major errors result in increased patient morbidity and even mortality.

In addition to routine preoperative assessment, particular attention should be given to the problems listed in Box 27.1.

Box 27.1 Specific preoperative problems in abdominal surgery

- Fluid balance
- Electrolyte disorders
- Full stomach
- Accompanying disease(s)
- Airway assessment
- Drugs

Fluid balance is often difficult to assess. A patient presenting with emergency bowel obstruction may have up to 2–3 litres of fluid sequestered in the bowel. Even in elective bowel surgery, the bowel is prepared by the liberal use of enemas before surgery. These patients are invariably dehydrated unless care is taken to provide adequate preoperative intravenous hydration.

How to Survive in Anaesthesia: A Guide for Trainees, Fourth Edition.
Neville Robinson, George Hall and William Fawcett.
© 2012 John Wiley & Sons, Ltd. Published 2012 by John Wiley & Sons, Ltd.

Vomiting can lead to dehydration and is one of the many causes of electrolyte disturbances in these patients. Hypokalaemia must be corrected before surgery, to avoid the complications listed in Box 27.2.

Box 27.2 Complications of hypokalaemia

• Arrhythmias
• Potentiation of competitive neuromuscular blocking drugs
• Prolonged ileus
• Respiratory muscle weakness
• Decreased inotropism

A thorough assessment of the airway is mandatory, and patients at risk of regurgitation or aspiration should have a rapid sequence induction.

Some diseases of the gut, such as ulcerative colitis and Crohn's disease, are multisystem diseases in which the skin, joints, eyes, mouth and renal systems may be affected. These patients are often receiving steroid therapy, and appropriate steroid cover must be provided in the perioperative period. For most patients hydrocortisone 25 mg intravenously at induction followed by 100 mg intravenously/24 hours until oral therapy is restarted is sufficient. Occasionally, it is necessary to give more hydrocortisone to maintain immune suppression during an acute illness. For example, a patient receiving 60 mg prednisolone/day should receive an equivalent dose of hydrocortisone (60 mg × 4 = 240 mg).

The perioperative problems of abdominal surgery are shown on Box 27.3.

Box 27.3 Perioperative considerations in abdominal surgery

• Rapid sequence induction of anaesthesia
• Venous access
• Muscular relaxation
• Vagal responses to surgery
• Infection
• Position of the patient
• Drugs
• Body temperature
• Adjunct regional analgesia
• Haemorrhage + fluid therapy

Most abdominal surgery requires adequate muscular relaxation. Sudden traction of viscera can stimulate vagally mediated reflexes and result in a bradycardia. Bowel inflammation, perforation and obstruction can lead to septicaemia, and antibiotics such as gentamicin, cefuroxime and metronidazole are often given pre- and intraoperatively. Gentamicin, an aminoglycoside antibiotic, theoretically potentiates the action of competitive neuromuscular blocking drugs. It is obviously a rare occurrence, as the authors have not encountered this problem.

Patients in the Lloyd Davies position can suffer nerve damage to the legs, and these should be padded appropriately. The common peroneal nerve at the top of the fibula is particularly at risk, and foot drop may occur postoperatively. Access to the airway and the venous cannula is often difficult.

Certain drugs affect bowel motility. Opioids increase circular smooth muscle contractility of the gut and hence bowel tone, decreasing propulsive activity. Nitrous oxide distends gas-filled cavities such as the bowel. Neostigmine increases gastrointestinal motility, which may threaten an intestinal anastomosis. There is little evidence, however, that the routine use of neostigmine increases the rate of anastomotic leaks after major abdominal surgery.

Heat conservation in abdominal surgical patients is important. The exposure of the viscera to air at room temperature exacerbates heat lost by radiation and convection. Temperature losses > 0.5 °C/hour have been found, particularly when peritoneal lavage is used. Heat loss should be prevented with hot-air warming blankets, heat and moisture filters in the circuit, and the use of warming devices for intravenous fluids.

Regional anaesthetic techniques, such as epidural anaesthesia, are often used to provide intraoperative and postoperative analgesia. Major bowel surgery cannot be carried out with these techniques alone unless a block above T4 is achieved. Regional anaesthesia is commonly used to supplement general anaesthesia with controlled ventilation for major surgery. The integrity of the bowel anastomosis is critically important in abdominal surgery. An adequate circulating blood volume and arterial pressure must be maintained to ensure that blood flow to the gut is not compromised.

Particular postoperative problems are shown in Box 27.4.

Box 27.4 Specific postoperative problems in abdominal surgery

- Analgesia
- Fluid balance
- Oxygen therapy
- High-dependency nursing care

Pain after laparotomy can result in hypoventilation, lung collapse and infection. Good postoperative analgesia is important, and regional anaesthesia is often used. Patient-controlled analgesia and subcutaneous opioid infusions are alternative techniques.

Careful fluid balance is important, as an ileus postoperatively can cause large fluid losses that are not recognised. Meticulous attention to urine output (> 0.5 ml/kg/h) and central venous and arterial pressure measurement will detect postoperative dehydration.

Intrapulmonary shunts and hypoventilation after abdominal surgery are common and may persist for up to 72 hours after surgery. Postoperative oxygen therapy may be needed during this time.

Appropriate nursing care must be provided after major abdominal surgery. This usually necessitates admission to a high dependency unit or intensive care unit.

Case study

An 84-year-old man presents with 6 days of abdominal pain. He is scheduled for a laparotomy with a diagnosis of perforated diverticular disease.

Preoperative care

Preoperative preparation is key to a successful outcome. The patient is likely to be dehydrated, haemoconcentrated with a very poor cardiac output and a metabolic acidosis. Time spent ensuring that the patient is as well resuscitated as possible is crucial. Apart from any comorbidities, the major issues are ensuring adequacy of circulation and treatment of sepsis. The patient will need oxygen, arterial and central venous access, possibly nasogastric tube and urinary catheter. Appropriate antibiotics are required. Investigations should include haemoglobin, urea and electrolytes, coagulation, and arterial blood gas analysis. Severe acidosis (base excess below −10 mmol/l) with a high lactate value has a poor prognosis. Before theatre the patient should be cardiovascularly stable, with good perfusion, urine output of 0.5 ml/kg/h and not acidotic. A CVP of around 8 mm Hg is ideal. Do not be pressurised by surgeons to anaesthetise a patient who is inadequately resuscitated. An hour or two in theatres optimising these patients before surgery improves outcome.

Perioperative care

Induction. Empty the stomach via the nasogastric tube. Rapid sequence induction. Cardiovascular decompensation is common. An epidural can be hazardous – sepsis, hypovolaemia, potential coagulopathy.

Maintenance. Scrupulous attention to fluid balance – patient may need inotropes if blood pressure falls in spite of a high CVP (> 10 mm Hg). Cardiac output measurement is helpful (e.g. oesophageal Doppler).

Postoperative care

Oxygen and pain control. Prolonged surgery, severe sepsis requiring inotropes and severe acidosis are indications for transfer to HDU/ICU for ventilation. Often these patients deteriorate significantly immediately after surgery.

27.2 Anal surgery

Operations in the anal region, such as anal stretch, drainage of perianal abscess, excision of pilonidal sinus, haemorrhoidectomy and lateral sphincterotomy can cause anaesthetic difficulties.

The surgeon often asks that the anal sphincter tone is not altered, and this precludes techniques using muscle relaxants and epidural, spinal and caudal anaesthesia, as they all relax the anal sphincter. These operations are short in duration but very painful. Profound anaesthesia is necessary, but the patient must awaken rapidly after surgery and be pain-free. A regional technique applied at the end of surgery, such as local anaesthetic infiltration or caudal anaesthesia, is helpful.

The anaesthetic problems of anal surgery are shown in Box 27.5.

Box 27.5 Anaesthetic problems of anal surgery

- Normal anal sphincter tone
- Depth of anaesthesia
- Intraoperative analgesia
- Position of patient
- Arrhythmias
- Laryngospasm
- Postoperative analgesia

The patient is usually placed in the lithotomy position; access to the venous cannula and airway may be difficult. If the depth of general anaesthesia is inadequate, arrhythmias, especially bradycardia, and laryngospasm may occur with the application of a painful stimulus. The anaesthetic therefore requires skill and simplicity. Anaesthesia is conducted with a suitable induction agent, opioid, and nitrous oxide, oxygen and a volatile agent. Atropine and suxamethonium *must* be available.

It is embarrassing for a previously smooth anaesthetic to degenerate into a noisy shambles as the patient develops laryngospasm when the haemorrhoid is clamped firmly by the surgeon. The management of laryngospasm is discussed in Chapter 18.

27.3 Conclusion

Major abdominal surgery is difficult. The patients are often ill, with pre-existing fluid and electrolyte problems. Careful preoperative assessment and resuscitation, and high-quality postoperative care, are essential.

A combination of general and regional anaesthesia is often appropriate. Beware anal surgery – a small orifice that causes big problems (anaesthetically, of course).

Chapter 28 Anaesthesia for dental and ENT surgery

The problems of anaesthetising for surgical procedures in and near the airway are common to both dental and ENT surgery.

28.1 Shared airway

A patent, secure airway is essential for safe anaesthetic practice. If possible, the tracheal tube or laryngeal mask airway should not protrude into the surgical field. Access to the airway is lost once the patient is draped and surgery started. The anaesthetic circuit is often long (and occasionally bulky), as the anaesthetic machine is placed at the feet of the patient. Two major problems may arise:
- The weight of the circuit can pull out or kink the tracheal tube: care must be taken to ensure that the circuit is supported to avoid drag.
- The surgeon may obstruct the tracheal tube when operating.

If the airway is lost, surgery must be stopped and appropriate adjustments made. Most surgeons understand the problems of the shared airway and are cooperative. However, one author had the alarming experience of the surgeon suddenly handing him the tracheal tube because it was interfering with the surgery.

Venous access is also restricted, and extension tubing on an intravenous cannula is essential.

28.2 Dental anaesthesia

Anaesthesia in the dental chair had a justifiable reputation as one of the major sporting events in anaesthetic practice. At present, dental anaesthesia is conducted either in hospital or in fully equipped premises, usually as

How to Survive in Anaesthesia: A Guide for Trainees, Fourth Edition.
Neville Robinson, George Hall and William Fawcett.
© 2012 John Wiley & Sons, Ltd. Published 2012 by John Wiley & Sons, Ltd.

day-stay surgery. The problems of dental anaesthesia are the same, irrespective of the place and duration of surgery. Dental operations can take only a few seconds, but you must provide suitable anaesthesia in an appropriate, safe environment.

There are many possible anaesthetic techniques for dental surgery (Box 28.1).

Box 28.1 Anaesthetic techniques for dental surgery

- Local anaesthesia
- Local anaesthesia and sedation
- Sedation
  - intravenous
  - inhalational
- General anaesthesia
- General anaesthesia and local anaesthesia

The teeth are supplied by branches of the trigeminal nerve, and dental surgeons are adroit at blocking the superior and inferior alveolar nerves at specific sites. Dental surgeons use prilocaine with adrenaline (epinephrine) or felypressin (a less toxic vasoconstrictor than adrenaline). If sedation is used, the patient must be able to talk to the anaesthetist or dental surgeon. Intravenous benzodiazepines are used frequently to provide sedation; occasionally Entonox (50% N_2O : 50% O_2) is inhaled.

There are many important considerations for general anaesthesia in dental surgery (Box 28.2).

Box 28.2 Considerations for general anaesthesia in dental surgery

- Antisialogogue
- Method of induction
- Type of tracheal tube
- Throat packs
- Surgical infiltration of local anaesthetic with felypressin
- Patient position – usually supine
- Mouth props
- Maintenance of anaesthesia
- Haemorrhage
- Arrhythmias

- Postoperative analgesia
- Laryngospasm
- Antibiotics
- Decrease in local swelling with steroids

Surgeons prefer a dry mouth, as it makes surgery easier. An anticholinergic drug in the premedication also protects against a bradycardia that often occurs during surgery. An intravenous induction is used if there are no difficulties with the airway. Control of the airway is obtained with a nasotracheal tube, and throat packs are inserted before surgery to collect blood and debris. It is easy to inadvertently leave the throat packs in at the end of surgery – obstruction of the airway occurs. One author always ties one end of the pack to the nasotracheal tube, or circuit, to act as an obvious reminder.

Complications during and after dental surgery are common. Severe haemorrhage is fortunately rare after dental surgery, but if there is any doubt about the adequacy of haemostasis then the patient must be kept in hospital under close observation. Arrhythmias are common (30% of patients) and can continue in the postoperative period. Oedema can be minimised by the use of steroids before surgery. Extubation of the trachea can be undertaken under light or deep anaesthesia. Under deep anaesthesia the patient is less likely to develop laryngospasm, but is more likely to aspirate vomit, blood or debris. Under light anaesthesia the patient has adequate protective reflexes, but is more prone to laryngospasm. We prefer the latter technique.

Emergency dental anaesthesia

Emergency dental anaesthesia should not be underestimated; get help from senior anaesthetists. The principal problem in a patient with a dental abscess or mandibular fracture is difficulty in opening the mouth, and hence with intubation. Distorted facial anatomy compounds the problem. Fibreoptic laryngoscopy and intubation is often necessary in these patients. Muscle relaxants must not be given until patency and control of the airway is secured.

Vigorous antibiotic therapy may decrease the infection, and the urgency of the surgery should be discussed with the dental surgeon. Only rarely is it a life-threatening emergency. If the airway is not safe postoperatively, the patient should be managed in the HDU.

Case study

A 23-year-old man with type 1 diabetes presents with a massive dental abscess. He has severe trismus, a blood glucose of 21 mmol/l and ketonuria.

Preoperative care
Control the severe hyperglycaemia with a glucose–insulin–potassium infusion and correct dehydration. Check circulating glucose and potassium.

Perioperative care
Induction. Choice of fibreoptic intubation, awake or sedated, or IV induction with nasal intubation (only for experienced anaesthetists). Avoid oral intubation if possible.
Maintenance. Fluids, antibiotics, aim for blood glucose < 10 mmol/l.

Postoperative care
Maintain glucose–insulin–potassium until oral intake resumed and then revert to usual insulin regimen. May require additional insulin until infection resolved.

28.3 ENT anaesthesia

The trainee is frequently introduced to anaesthesia for children on ENT lists. The anaesthetic problems of a child undergoing tonsillectomy and adenoidectomy are shown in Box 28.3.

Box 28.3 Anaesthetic considerations for tonsillectomy

- Child – problems with parents
- Premedication
- Induction of anaesthesia
- Type of tracheal tube
- Use of Boyle Davis gag
- Postoperative analgesia
- Laryngospasm
- Postoperative haemorrhage

A child with anxious parents needs special support. The parents are often present in the anaesthetic room during the induction of anaesthesia, which is undertaken either by the inhalational or the intravenous route. Sedative premedication is helpful. Oral midazolam syrup, oral atropine and topical EMLA cream are used commonly. A preformed tracheal tube (commonly a RAE tube) minimises, but does not exclude, the risk of the Boyle Davis gag kinking and obstructing the tube. Analgesia is given intravenously during surgery to decrease pain on emergence from anaesthesia. As in dental surgery, extubation can be carried out with the patient lightly or deeply anaesthetised. Laryngospasm is again a hazard. Postoperative haemorrhage is always a potential problem (see below).

The bleeding tonsil

Haemorrhage after a tonsillectomy is a serious complication and senior assistance must be sought. The anaesthetic problems are summarised in Box 28.4.

Box 28.4 Anaesthetic problems in the bleeding tonsil

- Senior help essential
- Occult haemorrhage
- Full stomach
- Patient often hypovolaemic
- Resuscitation
- Repeated anaesthesia
- Method of induction
  - inhalation
  - intravenous
- Secure airway
- Postoperative care

There may not be much visible evidence of haemorrhage; often all the blood is swallowed. If this occurs the stomach can contain a large amount of coagulated blood. A nasogastric tube will not remove this blood and aggravates the traumatised pharynx; it should not be used. The patient may be hypovolaemic, and full, appropriate resuscitation must occur before surgery.

There is debate about the method of facilitating tracheal intubation. An inhalational induction, with the patient head-down in the left lateral position, maintains control of the airway at all times and any bleeding trickles out of the mouth under gravity. A rapid sequence induction may be unsafe if there is blood, or a haematoma, in the pharynx, since the airway may become obstructed before the trachea is intubated. Although we prefer the former method, we have not seen serious sequelae from a rapid sequence induction.

A patient who has received two anaesthetics in a short time and required resuscitation should be managed in the HDU or even ICU postoperatively.

28.4 Ear surgery

Minor endoscopic procedures on the ear are conducted with the patient breathing spontaneously through a well-secured and correctly positioned laryngeal mask. More complex middle ear or mastoid operations have special problems (Box 28.5).

Box 28.5 Anaesthetic considerations for middle ear surgery

- Sedative premedication
- Avoidance of preoperative tachycardia
- Shared airway
- Prolonged surgery
- Use of nitrous oxide
- Hypotensive anaesthesia
- Postoperative vomiting
- Postoperative analgesia

The patient should arrive in the anaesthetic room sedated and with a normal heart rate. The avoidance of a tachycardia makes hypotensive anaesthesia easier to achieve. Nitrous oxide diffuses into air-filled spaces and in some surgical procedures causes difficulties. Many anaesthetists avoid nitrous oxide for middle ear surgery. Postoperative vomiting can be severe, and potent antiemetics are essential.

Induced hypotension is often used in these patients to decrease haemorrhage and improve the surgical field under the operating microscope. It is only suitable for patients without major cardiovascular disease, and mean arterial pressures less than 60 mm Hg are unnecessary. The techniques available are shown in Box 28.6.

Box 28.6 Techniques for induced hypotension

- No obstruction to venous outflow
- No coughing or straining (increases venous pressure)
- Head-up tilt
- Use of intermittent positive pressure ventilation
- Intra-arterial monitoring essential
- Specific hypotensive drugs
  - labetalol
  - nitroprusside
  - nitroglycerine

28.5 Conclusion

Sharing the airway with the surgeon is exciting; it ensures the vigilance of the anaesthetist. It is very difficult for a dental or ENT surgeon to kill the patient, other than by obstructing or dislodging the tracheal tube. If control and patency of the airway is lost, move the surgeon **immediately** and sort out the problem.

Chapter 29 **Anaesthesia for orthopaedic surgery**

In the bad old days a trainee anaesthetist spent long hours in the evening and night watching young orthopaedic surgeons struggle with 'emergency' cases. Fortunately, it has been agreed that patients with, for example, hip fractures need their surgery performed as soon as practically possible, but in the safest environment. The National Confidential Enquiry into Patient Outcome and Death (NCEPOD) recommends that such surgery should not be carried out by inexperienced surgeons and anaesthetists in the night. This work should be done on designated trauma lists during the day by appropriately trained staff.

29.1 General considerations

The general considerations of anaesthesia for orthopaedic surgery are shown in Box 29.1.

Box 29.1 General considerations in orthopaedic anaesthesia

- Age
- Trauma or elective
- Concomitant injury or disease
- Use of tourniquet
- Infection
- Haemorrhage
- Methylmethacrylate cement
- Deep vein thrombosis prophylaxis
- Fat embolism

How to Survive in Anaesthesia: A Guide for Trainees, Fourth Edition.
Neville Robinson, George Hall and William Fawcett.
© 2012 John Wiley & Sons, Ltd. Published 2012 by John Wiley & Sons, Ltd.

The extremes of the age range appear for orthopaedic surgery. Young people present commonly with trauma, while elderly patients often present for joint arthroplasty or with a fractured femoral neck. Age is not a contraindication to surgery, and you should learn to assess patients in terms of their *biological* age and not *chronological* age. Providing there are no major medical problems, elderly patients with hip fractures should have surgery on the earliest available trauma list. Otherwise, bed rest is associated with weakness, confusion, chest infection and deep vein thrombosis, and recovery from the delayed surgery is prolonged. Postoperative mortality and morbidity remain high in these patients.

After major trauma, emergency surgery on patients with compound fractures is common. Associated spinal and neck injuries must be sought and appropriate treatment instituted before induction of anaesthesia. Traumatic injuries, such as fractured ribs and a fractured pelvis, are often associated with damage to abdominal viscera such as the spleen and liver.

Orthopaedic surgery in the elderly is usually complicated by concomitant diseases. Patients for joint arthroplasties may have medical problems such as rheumatoid arthritis. Patients with hip fractures may simply have tripped and fallen, but the fall may have followed a cerebral ischaemic attack or a cardiac arrhythmia. Even carpal tunnel syndrome is sometimes associated with hypothyroidism, acromegaly and – in younger patients – pregnancy.

Tourniquets are used commonly to exsanguinate the limb and keep blood out of the operative field. They must be placed carefully to avoid creasing of the skin, which results in irritation and blister formation. Tourniquets are not used in people with sickle cell disease, for fear of provoking a sickle crisis. The recommended maximum duration of tourniquet time is 90 minutes. Pressures used are 33–40 kPa (250–300 mm Hg) for the arm and 46–53 kPa (350–400 mm Hg) for the leg. They must be fixed securely to prevent loosening. Haemorrhage after release of the tourniquet can be brisk. Red cell transfusion is usual after major traumatic fractures, but is now less common during and after joint arthroplasties.

The cement used in orthopaedic surgery is methylmethacrylate. This liquid monomer becomes a solid polymer after reconstitution, and heat is generated. The bone cavity should be vented as the cement is inserted to prevent embolism of bone marrow and debris. Occasionally severe hypotension occurs as the cement is inserted, although the precise mechanism is unknown. Extra vigilance is required at this time; the hypotension usually responds to the rapid administration of intravenous fluid. Occasionally vasopressors are required.

Deep vein thrombosis remains the cause of significant morbidity and mortality after orthopaedic surgery. Heparin prophylaxis is essential for major lower limb surgery.

Fat embolism occurs occasionally after trauma or surgery involving the pelvis or long bones (0.5–2% of patients). The initial symptoms and signs are as those of pulmonary thromboembolism. Fatty acid release causes diminished mental status, hypoxaemia, petechial haemorrhages and disseminated intravascular coagulation.

29.2 Anaesthesia for specific operations

Arm surgery

Arm surgery can be carried out under regional anaesthesia, general anaesthesia or a combination of both. The indications and contraindications of each technique need to be considered, together with the wishes of the patient and the surgeon. Anaesthetic considerations and techniques are shown in Box 29.2.

Box 29.2 Anaesthetic considerations and techniques for arm surgery

- Intravenous access
- Use of tourniquet
- Duration of surgery
- Concomitant diseases
- Patient preference
- Surgeon preference
- Emergency or elective
- Regional anaesthesia ± sedation
  - brachial plexus block
  - individual nerve blocks at elbow
  - local anaesthetic injection at operative site
- General anaesthesia
  - ? tracheal intubation
  - spontaneous ventilation or controlled ventilation

Regional anaesthesia avoids the drowsiness, nausea and vomiting of general anaesthesia, but can be difficult to perform, is slow in onset, and occasionally results in major complications such as pneumothorax and inadvertent intravascular injection (brachial plexus block). Nevertheless, if the patient and surgeon agree, we prefer regional rather than general anaesthesia.

Leg surgery

The anaesthetic considerations and techniques available for hip and knee surgery are shown in Box 29.3.

> **Box 29.3** Anaesthetic considerations and techniques for hip and knee surgery
>
> • Age
> • Elective or emergency surgery
> • Concomitant diseases
> • Patient position
> • Skin care
> • Nerve damage from positioning of patient
> • Haemorrhage
> • Infection
> • Methylmethacrylate cement
> • General anaesthesia
>   − spontaneous ventilation or controlled ventilation
> • Regional anaesthesia ± sedation
>   − spinal
>   − epidural
>   − femoral/sciatic nerve block
> • Combination of general and regional anaesthesia
> • Postoperative analgesia

Elderly patients have fragile skin which must be cared for appropriately. Nerve palsies can arise; suitable padding should be used.

The advantages and disadvantages of regional anaesthesia are shown in Box 29.4.

> **Box 29.4** Advantages and disadvantages of regional anaesthesia for hip and knee surgery
>
> • Advantages
>   − no risks from general anaesthesia
>   − decreased blood loss
>   − decreased risk of deep vein thrombosis
>   − better immediate postoperative analgesia
>   − earlier mobilisation
>   − decreased risk of respiratory infection
>   − less vomiting and mental confusion
> • Disadvantages
>   − surgeon preference
>   − patient preference

- complications of technique used
- hypotension
- headache
- difficult to perform in elderly

The advantages and disadvantages of general anaesthesia for hip surgery are shown in Box 29.5.

Box 29.5 Advantages and disadvantages of general anaesthesia for hip and knee surgery

- Advantages
  - often faster induction
  - patient preference
  - surgeon preference
  - better control of cardiovascular system
  - control of airway
  - avoids complications of regional anaesthesia
- Disadvantages
  - risks of general anaesthesia
  - slower recovery
  - slower mobilisation
  - more vomiting and confusion
  - increased risk of respiratory infection

We prefer regional anaesthesia, often combined with general anaesthesia, because of the decreased blood loss, decreased incidence of deep vein thrombosis and better analgesia after surgery.

Case study

A 79-year-old woman is scheduled for a cemented hemiarthroplasty following a fall.

Preoperative care

Ensure fully resuscitated. Patients often lose more than 500 ml of blood from a fracture. What was the reason for the fall? Take careful history, examination. Investigations should include ECG and haemoglobin, urea and electrolytes. Exclude cardiac/neurological cause for fall. Coexisting medical problems may need to be treated, but remember that better outcome is associated with early surgery. Delaying surgery may be counterproductive.

Perioperative care
Induction. Choice of regional or general anaesthetic, but may be difficult to position patient for regional block.
Maintenance. Ensure blood pressure and temperature maintained. May occasionally need invasive monitoring. Keep careful record of blood loss.

Postoperative care
Oxygen and good pain control. Early mobilisation.

Spinal surgery
Special considerations apply to anaesthesia for spinal surgery (Box 29.6).

Box 29.6 Anaesthetic considerations for spinal surgery

- Prone position
- Care of eyes
- Type of tracheal tube
- Difficult airway access – secure tube
- Difficult intravenous access
- Correct position of abdomen
- Specific nerve damage
- Infection
- Postoperative analgesia

Patients are usually prone, and corneal abrasions and pressure on the eyes must be prevented. The tracheal tubes used are nylon-reinforced to allow bending without kinking. They often need an introducer for insertion and, as they cannot be cut to a suitable size, may inadvertently pass into the right main bronchus. The tracheal tube must be well secured, as dislodgement when the patient is prone can be disastrous. The patient must be positioned correctly, often with the use of a Montreal mattress to support the chest and prevent compression of the abdomen. Abdominal compression decreases blood flow in the vena cava, but increases flow through the epidural veins, making surgery more difficult and increasing blood loss. Nerves liable to damage include the brachial plexus, ulnar nerves, nerves at the wrist and the femoral nerves. These must be padded appropriately. These operations are often painful, and appropriate postoperative analgesia must be given and discussed preoperatively with the patient. Regional anaesthesia is particularly effective but disliked by many surgeons as it interferes with neurological assessment.

29.3 Conclusion

Trauma and degenerative arthritic disease will ensure that orthopaedic surgery is not going to disappear. Much orthopaedic anaesthesia can be conducted with regional techniques; it is an excellent environment in which to learn these skills. Remember that orthopaedic surgeons are usually 'Black & Decker' men and sometimes have only a passing acquaintance with medicine.

Chapter 30 **Anaesthesia for day case surgery**

The assessment of day case patients is usually straightforward and is often delegated to senior nurses and new trainees. Surgeons frequently consider only the duration of surgery when deciding whether an operation can be undertaken on a day case basis. Their ability to ignore serious, chronic medical problems must never be underestimated. Most units have strict guidelines about the selection of patients for surgery as day cases. The most important considerations are the medical status of the patient, the potential surgical complications and the implications and side effects of anaesthesia. Typical selection guidelines are shown in Box 30.1.

Box 30.1 Selection guidelines for day case surgery

- Medical: ASA 1 and 2 only
  - age > 2 years < 80 years
  - obesity: BMI < 30
- Surgical: operating time < 60 minutes
  - minor and intermediate procedures
  - exclude procedures with significant postoperative pain
  - exclude procedures with significant risk of bleeding
  - exclude procedures with resultant significant disability
- Anaesthetic: no previous anaesthetic difficulties
- Social: must live within 10 miles/1 hour of hospital
  - must not go home by public transport
  - must have a responsible, fit escort
  - must be supervised by a responsible fit adult for 24 hours

---

In essence, the purpose of the guidelines is to ensure that relatively simple surgery with minimal complications is undertaken on healthy patients.

How to Survive in Anaesthesia: A Guide for Trainees, Fourth Edition.
Neville Robinson, George Hall and William Fawcett.
© 2012 John Wiley & Sons, Ltd. Published 2012 by John Wiley & Sons, Ltd.

Day case units are often isolated from the rest of the hospital and may not be equipped and staffed to the same standards as the main theatre complex. Provisions must be available to admit the occasional day case patient who has anaesthetic or surgical complications. After routine surgery the key decision is when to discharge the patient, and suitability is often assessed by the criteria shown in Box 30.2.

Box 30.2 Discharge criteria for day case surgery

- Stable vital signs for 1 hour after surgery
- No evidence of respiratory depression
- Orientated to person, place and time (or return to preoperative status)
- Ability to maintain oral fluids
- Ability to pass urine (particularly after regional anaesthesia)
- Able to dress (consistent with preoperative status)
- Able to walk (consistent with preoperative status)
- Minimal pain
- Minimal nausea and vomiting
- Minimal surgical bleeding
- Suitable escort present
- Written instructions for postoperative care

These criteria have been further developed in some units with the adoption of scoring systems to minimise subjective bias (Table 30.1).

Table 30.1 Discharge scoring criteria

Check	Result	Points
Vital signs	within 20% preoperative values	2
	within 20–40% preoperative values	1
	outside 40% preoperative values	0
Activity/mental status	orientated × 3 *and* steady gait	2
	orientated × 3 *or* steady gait	1
	neither	0
Pain/nausea/vomiting	minimal	2
	moderate, needed treatment	1
	severe, needs treatment	0
Surgical bleeding	minimal	2
	moderate	1
	severe	0
Intake/output	taken oral fluids *and* voided	2
	taken oral fluids *or* voided	1
	neither	0

Score ≥ 8 – fit for discharge
Score < 8 – unfit, medical assessment needed

30.1 Conclusion

Careful assessment of the patient presenting for day case surgery is essential to spot the medical problems missed by the surgeons. Adherence to the local selection guidelines should ensure a trouble-free anaesthetic, operation and recovery. However, do not expect all patients to obey instructions.

One author anaesthetised a local GP for a minor surgical procedure who discharged himself at noon to ride a motorcycle home for a light lunch before taking afternoon surgery!

Chapter 31 **Management of the patient in the recovery area**

At the end of surgery, the patient is usually transferred to the recovery area and is looked after by trained staff. Occasionally the patient needs to go to HDU/ICU, and this should be planned whenever possible. Last-minute requests for beds in HDU/ICU are deservedly unpopular. Do not transfer the patient from theatre if ventilation, circulation and neuromuscular function are inadequate. The operating theatre/anaesthetic room is a much safer environment for the patient than a long hazardous journey to recovery. Exhortations by surgeons and theatre staff to move the patient should be ignored until the patient is stable physiologically. All patients must be transferred from theatre to recovery breathing oxygen. Most recovery units accept patients with laryngeal mask airways still *in situ*, but tracheal tubes should only be left in place in exceptional circumstances (usually when IPPV is necessary).

The anaesthetist must explain what specific care is required in addition to the routine observations. The patient remains the responsibility of the anaesthetist during this time, and an anaesthetist must be available immediately should any problems arise. If you have any doubts about leaving the patient in the care of the recovery staff, then you must remain with the patient. This is essential if the patient is still intubated. Your duty lies with the patient you have just anaesthetised – the remaining cases have to wait.

The equipment and monitoring facilities in the recovery room should be the same as in a fully equipped operating theatre.

The objectives of care in the recovery room are shown in Box 31.1.

Box 31.1 Main objectives of care in the recovery area

- Assessment of conscious level
- Management of the airway
- Pain control

How to Survive in Anaesthesia: A Guide for Trainees, Fourth Edition.
Neville Robinson, George Hall and William Fawcett.
© 2012 John Wiley & Sons, Ltd. Published 2012 by John Wiley & Sons, Ltd.

- Essential monitoring and observation
- Avoidance of nausea and vomiting
- Management of shivering
- Temperature control
- Care of intravenous infusion
- Observation of surgical wound drainage
- Observation of urine output
- Oxygen therapy

Most units have guidelines on routine monitoring in the recovery area, and you must be familiar with them. One member of staff per patient is mandatory in the early postoperative period. Essential monitoring consists of careful clinical observation, and regular measurement of heart rate, arterial pressure, respiration and oxygen saturation. These measurements may be taken as frequently as every 5 minutes after major surgery, but at intervals of 15 minutes following routine minor surgery. In most units 'routine postoperative care' means recording the vital signs every 15 minutes. It may be desirable to monitor the patient by means of invasive techniques, such as arterial and central venous cannulation, and suitable equipment should be available in the recovery area.

31.1 Oxygen therapy

Oxygen therapy is often given routinely in the postoperative period, as hypoxaemia is an inevitable consequence of major surgery. The main causes of early postoperative hypoxaemia are shown in Box 31.2. However, hypoxaemia can persist for several days.

Box 31.2 Causes of early postoperative hypoxaemia

- Hypoventilation
  - airway obstruction
  - central respiratory depression
  - respiratory muscle weakness
- Ventilation/perfusion abnormalities
- Increased oxygen consumption
  - shivering
- Impaired response to hypoxaemia

> • Decreased oxygen content
>   – low cardiac output
>   – low haemoglobin values

Diffusion hypoxia is a transient phenomenon that occurs at the end of anaesthesia when nitrous oxide is replaced by air. Nitrous oxide enters the alveoli from the blood very rapidly. Because nitrogen is much less soluble than nitrous oxide, expired volume exceeds inspired volume, and there is a dilutional effect on oxygen in the alveoli.

The main causes of early postoperative hypoxaemia are a degree of *airway obstruction*, central respiratory depression usually caused by opioids, and respiratory muscle weakness resulting from inadequate reversal of neuro-muscular blocking drugs. Ventilation/perfusion abnormalities can arise after prolonged general anaesthesia and are exacerbated by factors such as obesity and pulmonary disease. Even very low concentrations of volatile anaesthetic agents impair the ventilatory response to hypoxaemia.

Oxygen is administered usually by a mask, either a fixed-performance or variable-performance device.

Fixed-performance oxygen masks

These masks provide an accurate inspired oxygen concentration which is independent of the patient's ventilation because the flow rate of fresh gas delivered is higher than the patient's inspiratory flow rate. They work on the principle of high air flow with oxygen enrichment (HAFOE). Air is entrained in oxygen by means of the Venturi principle to provide accurate concentrations of 24%, 28%, 35%, 40% and 60% oxygen, depending on which mask is used. The flow rates of oxygen required for these concentrations are written on the side of each mask. Such masks, for example the Ventimask, are expensive but are indicated when a precise concentration of oxygen needs to be given, such as in chronic obstructive lung disease. Following routine anaesthesia, cheaper, variable-performance masks are used.

Variable-performance oxygen masks

Variable-performance masks, such as the Hudson mask, depend on the pa-tient's inspiratory flow rate, the oxygen flow rate, and the duration of the expiratory pause. Nasal cannulae function in a similar way. If a patient is breathing normally then an oxygen flow of 4 litres/minute will provide an inspired oxygen concentration of about 40%. If necessary, this can be checked with an oxygen analyser.

If an inspired oxygen concentration of more than 60% is required, it cannot usually be given by a disposable oxygen mask. An anaesthetic face mask is necessary.

31.2 Calls from recovery

You will often be called to recovery to assess patients. In addition to the immediate problems such as airway obstruction and failure to breathe (see Chapter 19), the difficulties summarised in Box 31.3 are common and delay discharge of the patient to the ward.

Box 31.3 Delayed recovery problems

- Hypotension
  - common causes
    - bleeding and/or inadequate IV fluids
    - regional anaesthesia – epidural or spinal
    - left ventricular failure
    - vasodilation on rewarming
  - treatment: IV fluids (colloid) ± vasopressor
- Hypertension
  - common causes
    - pre-existing hypertension
    - pain
    - anxiety (secondary to inadequate reversal)
  - treatment: vasodilator, analgesia, reversal drugs
- Pain
  - consider the use of a variety of different drugs (multimodal analgesia) including
    - paracetamol IV
    - NSAIDs IV and PR
    - opioids (one route only)
    - local anaesthestics (top up epidural or nerve blocks if indicated)

Finally, recovery staff may chase you to complete inadequate anaesthetic charts and prescriptions for postoperative IV fluids, analgesics, antiemetics and oxygen. Their attention to detail may save your patients, your anaesthetic colleagues and the hospital legal department from major problems, so listen to their concerns, smile and do the needful.

31.3 Discharge

Criteria for discharge from the recovery room are becoming common. The main points of anaesthetic relevance are shown in Box 31.4.

Box 31.4 Typical criteria for discharge from recovery

- Patient awake and responds appropriately to commands
- Upper airway patent and reflexes present
- Respiration satisfactory
- Cardiovascular stability
- Pain control adequate, not vomiting
- Normothermic
- Analgesics, antiemetics, IV fluids, oxygen prescribed

31.4 Conclusion

The care of the patient in the recovery room remains the responsibility of the anaesthetist, who must be available to deal with any complications that may arise. The anaesthetist is also responsible for the discharge of the patient from the recovery area to the ward, and increasingly this is a formal, documented procedure. Remember that the recovery room is a good refuge for patients who need resuscitation before surgery – the staff are usually on your side.

Chapter 32 **Postoperative analgesia**

Pain is a subjective response to noxious stimuli, and patients vary greatly in their need for analgesia after surgery. For example, the amount of morphine requested postoperatively varies tenfold after the same operation. Analgesic regimens must take into account this unpredictable response. Acute pain teams are a popular development in anaesthetic practice and have drawn attention to past failings in the provision of adequate postoperative analgesia. The advantages claimed for good analgesia are shown in Box 32.1.

Box 32.1 Claimed advantages of good postoperative analgesia

- Humanitarian reasons
- Psychological reasons
- Fewer respiratory complications
- Fewer adverse cardiovascular responses
- Fewer autonomic complications (sweating, vomiting)
- Earlier mobilisation
- Less deep vein thrombosis
- Earlier return to normal life style/work

The humanitarian and psychological advantages of good analgesia are obvious. Pain, especially after abdominal surgery, can lead to deterioration in respiratory function from a reduction in ventilatory capacity and an inability to cough. Pulmonary atelectasis and infection are more likely. Pain causes tachycardia and hypertension, and this may exacerbate any existing myocardial ischaemia. Sweating and vomiting may accompany pain, and good analgesia makes early mobilisation and rehabilitation easier.

How to Survive in Anaesthesia: A Guide for Trainees, Fourth Edition.
Neville Robinson, George Hall and William Fawcett.
© 2012 John Wiley & Sons, Ltd. Published 2012 by John Wiley & Sons, Ltd.

32.1 Influences on postoperative pain

Postoperative pain is affected by many factors, including those listed in Box 32.2.

Box 32.2 Factors influencing postoperative pain

- Age
- Sex
- Social class
- Anxiety
- Understanding of surgery
- Attitudes of staff
- Pain relief in other patients
- Type of surgery
- Type of anaesthesia

The elderly tolerate pain better than younger adults, and women are more stoical than men. People in social classes III, IV and V tolerate pain better than those in social classes I and II. Patients with a high preoperative neuroticism score experience more pain. A reduction in anxiety and education of the patient about the surgery have been shown to decrease postoperative pain.

The attitudes of staff and the adequacy of analgesia provided for other patients on the ward are also important. Staff who are reluctant, or have little time to provide good postoperative analgesia, adversely affect the patient's recovery. Fear of the side effects of drugs (for example, addiction to opioids) is a totally unacceptable reason for the nursing staff not providing as much analgesic as required.

32.2 Methods of postoperative analgesia

An approach to the postoperative analgesic requirements of the patient must be considered during the preoperative visit (Box 32.3).

Box 32.3 General plan of postoperative analgesia

- Preoperative assessment and discussion with patient
- Premedication
- Systemic drugs
  - non-steroidal anti-inflammatory drugs

- opioids
- route
  - oral
  - intramuscular
  - intravenous
  - subcutaneous
  - rectal
- mode of administration
  - patient-controlled or by medical staff
  - continuous versus intermittent methods
- Regional anaesthetic techniques
  - local anaesthetic agent
  - addition of opioid
  - route
    - epidural
    - spinal
    - caudal
    - specific nerve blocks
    - wound infiltration
  - mode of administration
    - single bolus at surgery/intermittent/infusion
- Miscellaneous techniques
  - steroids
  - Entonox
  - transcutaneous nerve stimulation
  - acupuncture
- Benefits versus side effects
- Follow-up

The importance of the preoperative visit and explanation to the patient of the procedures cannot be overemphasised. Consent for unusual routes of drug administration (for example, rectal in the UK) must be obtained. In some patients postoperative analgesia starts with premedication and the administration of opioids.

Systemic drugs
Non-steroidal anti-inflammatory drugs (NSAIDs) such as aspirin, paracetamol, diclofenac and piroxicam can be given as oral analgesics. These agents are often mixed with codeine and dihydrocodeine, which are occasionally

given by themselves. The choice of drugs depends on the personal preference of the anaesthetist. NSAIDs have important side effects (Box 32.4).

Box 32.4 Main side effects of NSAIDs

• Gastric ulceration
• Decreased platelet aggregation
• Drug interactions (e.g. diuretics and serum potassium)
• Hypersensitivity
• Renal impairment

Morphine is the 'gold standard' opioid drug and is widely used for post-operative analgesia. Pethidine is claimed to be less sedative and have relaxant properties on smooth muscle. We consider pethidine to be a potent emetic and weak analgesic and never use it. All opioids have side effects (Box 32.5).

Box 32.5 Major side effects of systemic opioids

• Nausea and vomiting
• Sedation
• Dysphoria
• Euphoria
• Constipation
• Delayed stomach emptying
• Hallucinations

The traditional method of providing postoperative analgesia, by giving intramuscular morphine on request by the patient, has many drawbacks including intermittent analgesia and inadequate dosage.

Patient-controlled analgesia (PCA)

Syringe pumps have been devised so that the patients (not visitors, or members of staff) can administer their own analgesia intravenously. The pumps must be safe and programmed to provide sufficient analgesia after major surgery (Table 32.1). Once programmed they must be locked so that neither the syringe of opioid nor the controls are accessible. Patient-controlled analgesia does not mean patient-programmed analgesia. Careful explanation to the patient about PCA is essential for the success of the technique.

Table 32.1 Typical regimen for intravenous morphine PCA pump

Drug details	Regimen
Dose	50 mg in 50 ml sodium chloride
Concentration	1 mg/ml
Bolus dose	1 mg
Lock-out time	5 minutes
Hourly dose limit	12 mg

In theory, if patients become too drowsy they will not push the button and so will not receive excessive doses of opioid. Despite this, staff must monitor, at least hourly, the severity of the pain, the amount of analgesia used, the degree of sedation, and the respiratory rate. If the respiratory rate is less than 10 breaths/minute or the patient too drowsy, the infusion must be stopped. The opioid antagonist, naloxone, must be available and can be given in cases of severe respiratory depression, but it should be remembered that analgesia will also be reversed. Repeated small doses of naloxone may be necessary.

Subcutaneous infusions

Opioids can be administered subcutaneously by continuous infusion pumps that are altered by the staff, not the patient. Morphine is given at a concentration of 2.5 mg/ml (50 mg in 20 ml sodium chloride solution). For example, the infusion is given at a rate of 1.25–3.75 mg/h. Increments of 2.5 mg can be given for breakthrough pain. Monitoring must be undertaken as described above; overdose again causes severe drowsiness and respiratory depression.

Regional techniques

Local anaesthetic drugs can be administered as a single bolus, by intermittent injections, or as a continuous infusion. They can be given into the subcutaneous tissue around a wound, into joints, the pleural cavity, and in the region of the spinal cord (epidural, spinal, caudal). Opioids are often given by the epidural route, either in combination with local anaesthetics, or individually, to provide analgesia. Local anaesthetics have toxic side effects (see Chapter 15). The balance of possible complications versus benefits must be considered.

Miscellaneous

Entonox (50% N_2O : 50% O_2) is used to help alleviate the pain of short-lived procedures such as the removal of chest drains. Steroids can reduce swelling and consequently pain in dental procedures.

Transcutaneous nerve stimulators and acupuncture are used occasionally as adjuncts to other analgesic techniques.

32.3 Conclusion

Many techniques are currently available to provide pain relief after surgery. Side effects are inevitable, and some of these, such as vomiting with opioids, can be distressing. It is essential that you see the effectiveness or otherwise of the chosen postoperative analgesic regimen and ask the patients for their opinions.

Chapter 33 **Management of head injuries**

Patients with head injuries suffer *primary* brain damage at the time of the trauma. Secondary brain damage occurs after the initial insult and is caused by a decrease in cerebral perfusion and oxygenation. The anaesthetist can reduce morbidity and mortality from *secondary* brain damage by preventing or treating the causes listed in Box 33.1.

Box 33.1 Causes of secondary brain damage after trauma

- Hypoxaemia
- Hypercapnia
- Hypotension
- Increased cerebral venous pressure
  - coughing
  - straining
- Infection

33.1 General considerations

A rapid assessment of the patient must take place before resuscitation and treatment. Physical examination must include a careful assessment of the cervical spine, as there is a high correlation between skull fractures and neck fractures. The neck should be immobilised by in-line cervical traction, or a stiff neck collar, until radiographic exclusion of a fracture has been undertaken. Life-threatening chest and abdominal injuries should be looked for carefully, and control and treatment of these should take priority over transfer or neurosurgical intervention. Neurosurgical units are often isolated

---

How to Survive in Anaesthesia: A Guide for Trainees, Fourth Edition.
Neville Robinson, George Hall and William Fawcett.
© 2012 John Wiley & Sons, Ltd. Published 2012 by John Wiley & Sons, Ltd.

hospitals and have to transfer patients to nearby hospitals for major thoracic and abdominal surgery before neurosurgical intervention.

The airway must be cleared of blood, loose teeth and debris, and protected by tracheal intubation if necessary. Assessment of the airway is mandatory, and you should assume that the patient has a full stomach. If intubation is deemed necessary, and airway assessment shows that this is likely to be successful, then a rapid sequence induction technique can be undertaken. Thiopentone and propofol attenuate the rise in intracranial pressure that occurs with laryngoscopy. Suxamethonium increases intracranial pressure transiently, but this is acceptable compared with the risks of an obstructed airway. Furthermore, hyperventilation after intubation rapidly decreases intracranial pressure. A nasogastric tube empties the stomach, and should be inserted after tracheal intubation. The reasons for tracheal intubation in a patient with a head injury are shown in Box 33.2.

Box 33.2 Indications for tracheal intubation in the head-injured patient

• Airway protection
  - loss of laryngeal reflexes
  - unconscious patient (GCS < 8)
  - compromised airway (e.g. facial injuries)
• Hypoventilation
  - hypoxaemia
  - hypercapnia
  - associated chest injury
  - associated drugs
  - airway obstruction
  - aspiration of gastric contents
• Before interhospital transfer
  - neurological deterioration in transit
  - convulsions
  - unconscious patient (GCS < 8)

Hypoventilation causes hypoxia and hypercapnia, and coughing and straining on a tracheal tube increases intracranial pressure. Controlled hyperventilation to a P_aCO_2 of about 4 kPa is used to control intracranial pressure, and neuromuscular blocking drugs are given, if required. A $P_aO_2 \geq 13$ kPa should be achieved.

Hypotension results in reduced cerebral perfusion, and adequate fluid replacement is essential. Closed head injury is never a cause of hypotension in adults, and other factors must be sought.

Neurological assessment is undertaken with the Glasgow Coma Scale (GCS) (Table 33.1).

Table 33.1 The Glasgow Coma Scale (GCS): neurological assessment

Response	Score
Best motor response	
obeys commands	6
withdraws from painful stimuli	5
localises to painful stimuli	4
flexes to painful stimuli	3
extends to painful stimuli	2
no response	1
Best verbal response	
orientated	5
confused speech	4
inappropriate words	3
incomprehensible sounds	2
none	1
Eye opening response	
spontaneously	4
to speech	3
to pain	2
none	1

Localising signs and pupillary reaction should additionally be sought and noted. Sequential changes in GCS score are a convenient way of assessing neurological progress. A GCS less than 8 is serious, and often an indication for tracheal intubation.

Further management of the head-injured patient includes the use of intravenous mannitol (0.5 g/kg), which decreases intracranial pressure transiently. Anticonvulsants may be necessary if seizures occur, and antibiotics are used prophylactically in patients with compound skull fractures. Further advice can be obtained from the regional neurosurgical centre.

33.2 Interhospital transfer

Patients are often transferred for neurosurgery. The decision whether to operate or not depends on the CT scans of the brain.

Guidelines for transferring head-injured patients are shown in Box 33.3.

Box 33.3 Guidelines for transferring head-injured patients

- Physiological stabilisation before transfer
- Escorting doctor of adequate experience
- Appropriate drugs and equipment for transfer
- Intubated patients require
  - sedation
  - paralysis
  - analgesia if indicated
- Use short-acting drugs to allow neurological assessment
- Monitoring to minimal acceptable standard

Intubated patients should not increase intracranial pressure during transfer by coughing or straining, and hyperventilation is maintained. Short-acting drugs such as propofol, fentanyl and muscle relaxants are used. A detailed handover to the receiving anaesthetist at the neurosurgical centre is essential.

33.3 Conclusion

The anaesthetist has a major role in the management of the head-injured patient, and the prevention of any secondary brain damage is the initial priority. Transfer of a patient with a head injury to a neurosurgical centre is not supposed to be undertaken by a novice trainee. However, this still occurs frequently, and if you have any doubts about the airway and/or neurological state, tracheal intubation and ventilation should be undertaken.

Chapter 34 **Anaesthesia in the corridor**

Occasionally you will be asked to undertake anaesthesia away from the operating theatres. Inexperienced anaesthetists are not supposed to be involved with such work, as 'playing away from home' is more hazardous.

Within the hospital, anaesthetics may be given in:
- psychiatric unit for electroconvulsive therapy
- accident and emergency department
- coronary care unit
- radiology department

Outside the hospital you may be asked to maintain anaesthesia during the transfer of patients between hospitals.

The principles and practice of safe anaesthesia remain the same regardless of the site. The essential requirements are shown in Box 34.1, and, if these are not met, the patient should be transferred to a safe environment. A senior anaesthetist must be called if any anaesthetic difficulty is anticipated.

Box 34.1 Minimum requirements for conduct of anaesthesia

- Qualified, experienced assistance
- Checked anaesthetic machine
  - medical gas supplies
  - vaporisers
  - breathing systems
  - ventilator
- Adequate suction
- Adequate table tilt
- At least two working laryngoscopes
- Appropriate range of face masks, airways, tracheal tubes

How to Survive in Anaesthesia: A Guide for Trainees, Fourth Edition.
Neville Robinson, George Hall and William Fawcett.
© 2012 John Wiley & Sons, Ltd. Published 2012 by John Wiley & Sons, Ltd.

- Minimal monitoring equipment with alarms
- Appropriate drugs available
- Resuscitation drug box present
- Defibrillator working
- Appropriate recovery facilities and staff

In general, anaesthesia needing a rapid sequence induction should be carried out in the main operating theatres.

Crises and complications can occur anywhere, and you must be prepared. Do not be persuaded to work with inadequate facilities. Local medical staff can be very reassuring about the safety of anaesthesia over the last 20 years in some far corridor of the hospital.

34.1 Electroconvulsive therapy

Therapeutic convulsive therapy is used for the treatment of severe depression. The anaesthetist must consider the points shown in Box 34.2 in addition to the minimum requirements for the provision of anaesthesia.

Box 34.2 Considerations for electroconvulsive therapy anaesthesia

- Remote-site anaesthesia
- Mental state of patient
- Modified convulsion
- Teeth protection
- Concomitant drug therapy
- Short-duration procedure

After induction of anaesthesia, the convulsion is modified by the use of small doses of suxamethonium (25–50 mg), which makes the patient apnoeic for a few minutes. Muscle pain after anaesthesia is not a major problem. The teeth must be protected by a mouth guard when the convulsion is applied.

Since the anaesthetist must not touch the patient at the initiation of the convulsion, adequate oxygenation must be ensured before treatment.

34.2 Accident and emergency anaesthesia

The anaesthetist is a frequent visitor to the accident and emergency department to assist in cardiopulmonary resuscitation. Anaesthesia in this environment used to be common and was undertaken in difficult conditions; monitoring and recovery facilities were often non-existent. Two authors have been involved with 'casualty lists' – these were hazardous for the patients and apparently character-building for us.

Only if the basic requirements of safe anaesthesia are met (Box 34.1) should surgery occur. Anaesthesia is often challenging, for example for drainage of an abscess in an unpremedicated patient. If you have any doubt about the safety of the patient, surgery must be undertaken in the main operating theatres.

34.3 Radiological procedures

Again, the basic requirements of safe anaesthesia must be met. For scanning procedures, the anaesthetist often has to leave the patient and move to the scanning room, returning to monitor the patient physically between scans. You must be able to see the patient, either through a window or by remote television, at all times. The monitoring equipment must always be clearly visible. In radiological procedures, the anaesthetic circuit is often 2–3 m long, and access to the airway and venous cannula is difficult during scanning. General anaesthesia with control of the airway is nearly always safer than sedation. In particular, never sedate a patient with a head injury. Beware of the 'urgent' patient with abdominal bleeding who is sent for a CT scan before surgery – resuscitation in the x-ray department in the middle of the night is to be avoided at all costs.

34.4 Anaesthesia for cardioversion

Cardioversion is often undertaken in the coronary care unit, where appropriate monitoring is usually available. This avoids the risks of moving a sick patient. Any subsequent arrhythmias are usually managed by the cardiologist. The minimum requirements for safe anaesthesia must be met. Often the procedure is of short duration and the cardioversion occurs under the induction dose of the intravenous agent.

34.5 Interhospital transfer of patients

The monitoring requirements of patients undergoing anaesthesia were discussed in Chapter 10. Similar requirements must be met when patients are transferred. Additional anaesthetic considerations are shown in Box 34.3.

Box 34.3 Anaesthetic considerations for patient transfer

- Medical condition of patient needing transfer
- Familiarity with equipment
- Secure airway and vascular access
- Drugs to manage transfer safely
- Appropriate monitoring
- Transfer to a suitable member of staff at receiving hospital

---

Patients should be physiologically stable before transfer. Ambulances often contain ventilators and suction equipment that are different from those found in hospitals. Familiarisation with these is essential before the patient is moved. Tracheal tubes and intravenous cannulae must be secure. The correct drugs for the maintenance of anaesthesia, paralysis and resuscitation must be available. A ventilated patient requires the same monitoring as in theatre or the intensive care unit.

34.6 Ward work

You may be called to the surgical ward to help sort out problems after surgery. These calls often occur at unsocial hours, and the initial appraisal should follow the basic Airway Breathing Circulation. Do not attempt major resuscitation in the ward but move the patient to theatres/recovery unit.

Common problems on surgical wards are:
- Hypotension – this is often the result of blood loss, and an IV bolus of colloid will correct the problem. Remember other possibilities such as myocardial infarction, pulmonary embolus and sepsis.
- Loss of consciousness – this may result from the inappropriate administration of analgesics ± sedatives, particularly opioids, cerebrovascular accidents, hypo/hyperglycaemia and hypothyroidism.
- Epidural infusions – hypotension usually responds to an IV bolus of colloid, but a small dose of ephedrine may be necessary. Inadequate pain control can be difficult to manage. A small bolus (5–10 ml) from the pump may help, the catheter may need to be withdrawn so that only 3 cm are left in the epidural space, particularly if there is a unilateral block, or it may be possible to give an opioid epidurally *or* intravenously. Never give epidural and IV opioids simultaneously. If you are unsure, remove the epidural and use another method(s) of analgesia. The 'leaking' epidural usually needs resiting. Severe back pain and progressive weakness of the legs are fortunately rare but need urgent intervention. Stop

the epidural and if the problem does not resolve rapidly consider an epidural haematoma.

34.7 Conclusion

Beware of anaesthesia in some distant outpost of the hospital. If you have any doubts about the safety of the procedure, then insist that the patient is moved to the main operating theatres. Any inconvenience that this may cause is trivial when compared with the occurrence of an anaesthetic disaster.

Chapter 35 **Anaesthetic aphorisms**

If you cannot be bothered to read all the other chapters then the following aphorisms will teach you a lot about the safe practice of anaesthesia. We thank our anaesthetic colleagues, past and present, for their help in compiling this list of epigrams that includes wisdom, witticism and a large helping of the obvious.

35.1 General

- Never start an anaesthetic until you have seen the whites of the surgeon's eyes.
- Always pee before starting a list.
- If you are feeling tired the **three S's** is a good reviver – a shit, a shave and a shower (politically incorrect, but we do not know the female equivalent).
- ABC of anaesthesia – always be cool, always be cocky!
- ABCD of resuscitation – arrive, blame, criticise and depart.
- Remember **KISS** – **K**eep **I**t **S**imple, **S**tupid.
- Anaesthesia is 'awfully simple' but when it goes wrong is 'simply awful'.
- Always look carefully at previous anaesthetic charts.
- If in doubt, ask for help. There is no place for arrogance in anaesthesia.
- Big syringe, little syringe, white knob, blue knob, big purple knob – good for most things.
- First rule of anaesthesia – if there is a chair in theatre, sit on it.
- Preoperative assessment – always find out **who** is doing the operation, **what** time it is happening and **where** the patient is going after surgery.
- Accidents are funny things. You don't know they are happening until they happen (A. A. Milne). Stay vigilant.

How to Survive in Anaesthesia: A Guide for Trainees, Fourth Edition.
Neville Robinson, George Hall and William Fawcett.
© 2012 John Wiley & Sons, Ltd. Published 2012 by John Wiley & Sons, Ltd.

- Never panic. This applies particularly when the patient is trying to die and you have no idea why.
- Where there is cyanosis there is life – just!
- 99% of anaesthetics is dead easy. 1% is easy dead!

35.2 Airway

- If in doubt, take it out. This applies to tracheal tubes and many other things in life.
- There are three things to respect in anaesthesia – the airway, the airway and the airway.
- When all else fails, disconnect the catheter mount and blow down the tracheal tube.
- Careless 'torque' costs lives – don't let breathing tubes kink.
- The laryngoscope is a tongue retractor, not a tooth extractor.
- Nobody dies from failure to intubate the larynx, they die from failure to ventilate and oxygenate.
- The expired gas contains no carbon dioxide when you ventilate the stomach.
- Fix tracheal tubes as if your life depended on it – the patient's life does!
- The first five causes of sudden hypoxia in an intubated, ventilated patient are the tube, the tube, the tube, the tube, and finally the tube. The tracheal tube may be dislodged, disconnected, blocked or kinked, or the cuff herniated.
- If you anticipate a difficult airway, premedication with a drying agent is useful.
- In patients with a potentially difficult airway **always** have a plan B before starting anaesthesia.
- If you do have a problem with the airway, document it carefully for the next anaesthetist.
- Beware of patients with a beard – a receding chin may lurk beneath (this is strongly denied by one author).
- 'Sniffing the morning air' position for tracheal intubation can be described as the position of the head when taking the first sip from a pint of beer.
- The tip of a gum-elastic bougie can be bent after warming with hot tap water. If you try to bend it when cold, it will snap.
- Remember the humble nasopharyngeal airway. It is useful in patients with poor mouth opening, loose teeth and expensive dental work.

35.3 Cannulation

- Always keep the giving sets on the appropriate side of the patient (left arm, left side). If you don't, think what will happen when you move the patient – one out, all out.

- Use a 2 ml syringe to unblock a clotted cannula (basic physics).
- If the patient is going to ICU/HDU you will never have enough venous access – always insert a spare cannula.
- Over flat areas of skin, such as the forearm, a **slight** upward bend of the cannula makes insertion easier (if the bend is excessive the needle will not come out!).
- Never try to apply adhesive dressing with your gloves on (real men don't wear gloves).
- If you think that you might need invasive monitoring, you will. Insert the cannula.
- If you have to cannulate the brachial artery, rather than the radial artery, use a 5 cm long cannula rather than 3 cm to prevent kinking when the elbow flexes.
- If you are struggling to find a vein in the antecubital fossa, externally rotate the arm and look carefully on the medial aspect of the forearm.
- Twice the diameter of a cannula gives 16 times the flow rate. Never use a venous cannula smaller than 16 gauge.
- Never say to the patient 'just a little prick' before inserting a cannula – you are likely to be told that is exactly what you are!
- A Swan–Ganz introducer is the best cannula for massive haemorrhage.
- Never anaesthetise a woman of child-bearing age without inserting a large-bore venous cannula (? ectopic pregnancy).
- Put blood bags into pressure infusers with the label furthest from you. When you can see the label the bag is empty.

35.4 Monitoring and equipment

- Never use a ventilator, anaesthetic machine or any equipment with which you are unfamiliar. This is an **absolute** rule after hours.
- If you have a problem with the ventilator/breathing system that you cannot instantly identify and correct, change to a simple circuit and hand-ventilate the patient.
- Know where the defibrillator is kept in theatre and how it works.
- If a monitor gives an abnormal value, such as low oxygen saturation, check the patient and then the equipment.
- Make sure that you are not the only sucker in the anaesthetic room/theatre.
- An AMBU bag is invaluable in a power failure!

35.5 Regional anaesthesia

- Never persuade an unwilling patient to have regional anaesthesia.
- If you need midazolam/fentanyl with your local block, it has failed.

- When inserting an epidural catheter, thread it straight from the sterile bag to prevent it uncoiling and touching something unsterile.
- It is often easier in the elderly to insert the epidural/spinal with the patient in a sitting position, leaning forward.
- Try the L5/S1 interspace when you have failed higher up the spine.
- When using saline to identify the epidural space keep a small bubble of air at the top of the syringe. When there is no resistance to injection of saline into the epidural space, the bubble will not change shape until it reaches the bottom of the syringe.
- If it is difficult to thread an epidural catheter through the needle, withdraw the needle very slightly.

35.6 Drugs

- All 1 ml ampoules look the same – check very carefully.
- Always label all syringes.
- Atropine and adrenaline (epinephrine) are often stored next to each other.
- Suxamethonium can easily be given in error for all drugs found in 2 ml syringes.
- Thiopentone solution can look like augmentin, and antibiotics do not induce anaesthesia.
- Put the label on the syringe at the volume you fill it to. You can check later how much you have given.
- Intravenous drugs go into veins, so colour-code the three-way taps. Blue for venous, red for arterial. If the cannula has a filter it is in the epidural space!
- For a rapid sequence induction always have two doses of suxamethonium ready in case one goes over the floor/ceiling etc.

35.7 Conclusion

Anaesthesia is fun. We still enjoy it after a total of more than 90 years' practice. Remember:

- Be kind – patients are very vulnerable.
- Be prepared – plan your anaesthetic.
- Be professional – try to emulate Humphrey Bogart's definition of a professional as somebody who can still give their best performance when they feel least like it!

And finally . . .

If you have read this book you have the basics of safe anaesthetic practice. You will have difficulties and make mistakes – we all do. If you do not have problems then either you are not working hard or you are not being honest. Discuss your problems with other anaesthetists, never be afraid to ask for help (we still do), and try not to keep making the same mistake! If in doubt, keep it simple. A secure airway and good venous access are the key to safe anaesthesia.

Enjoy life – you have joined a great specialty.

Index

How to Survive in Anaesthesia: A Guide for Trainees, Fourth Edition.
Neville Robinson, George Hall and William Fawcett.
© 2012 John Wiley & Sons, Ltd. Published 2012 by John Wiley & Sons, Ltd.